MEN
and
AGING

Recent Titles in
Bibliographies and Indexes in Gerontology

MEN
and
AGING

———◆———

A Selected, Annotated Bibliography

Compiled by
Edward H. Thompson, Jr.

**Bibliographies and Indexes in Gerontology,
Number 32**

GREENWOOD PRESS
Westport, Connecticut • London

Library of Congress Cataloging-in-Publication Data

Thompson, Edward H.
   Men and aging : a selected, annotated bibliography / compiled by
Edward H. Thompson, Jr.
      p.   cm.—(Bibliographies and indexes in gerontology, ISSN
   0743–7560 ; no. 32)
      Includes indexes.
      ISBN 0–313–29106–3 (alk. paper)
      1. Aged men—Bibliography.   2. Middle aged men—Bibliography.
   I. Title.   II. Series.
   Z7164.04T5   1996
   [HQ1061]
   016.30526 s—dc20
   [016.3053]   95–25580

British Library Cataloguing in Publication Data is available.

Library of Congress Catalog Card Number: 95–25580
ISBN: 0–313–29106–3
ISSN: 0743–7560

First published in 1996

Greenwood Press, 88 Post Road West, Westport, CT 06881
An imprint of Greenwood Publishing Group, Inc.

Printed in the United States of America

∞™

The paper used in this book complies with the
Permanent Paper Standard issued by the National
Information Standards Organization (Z39.48–1984).

10 9 8 7 6 5 4 3 2 1

Contents

— ◆ —

Preface

— ♦ —

This book of annotations began several years back when I was rummaging for articles which could inform undergraduates about older men's lives. I had planned a pair of lectures for my undergraduates at Holy Cross College, one discussing the social worlds of older women and the next on older men. Preparation for the first lecture came easily, since a sizable literature on that half of the gender-by-late-life interaction already had been published. There were problems, however, when I turned to draw together the literature on older men. I found very little work which directly addressed older men's lives. I turned to what I anticipated was the quick rescue -- an electronic search of the medical, behavioral science, and social science literatures. When I keyed in the search "old men," the hit rate was near zero. The gender category "men" was not one that was listed, even though the category "women" was. I discovered, with the assistance of reference librarians, that to unearth materials on older men required using the key words "aged males" and then limiting the search to humans only, in order exclude several thousand articles on aged laboratory male rats. The electronic return signaled that better than 9,000 articles were available. I was relieved, until I discovered that virtually all of the articles were about aging and not older men.

I had the good fortune to benefit from these developments. Long before this book of annotations was conceived, I had asked Tony Stankus, the Science Librarian at Holy Cross, to run a preliminary search for me on identifying the social science and medical literatures on older men. He graciously jumped in but found little. He confirmed what I now suspected, namely that the literature on older men was sparse and not readily identifiable.

A year earlier, conversations and exchanges with colleagues at Case Western University, where I had been warmly included as a visiting associate professor for the fall semester while on a funded research leave from Holy Cross, proved to be the encouragement needed to take on this project. That semester immersed me into routine discussions about aging and gender. Sarah Matthews, whose office was in the same alcove, kept asking me these intriguing, pointed questions about issues of gender and age. Those questions were only part of her direct encouragement, for her earlier book on the *Social Worlds of Older Women* had long been on my bookshelf. Eva Kahana, whose office was around the corner, made me feel fully included. As Chair of the Department of Sociology, Eva mentored me in my temporary appointment. At least several times a week she would stop by my office to query about my week's work and to discuss concerns in gerontology. Those conversations with Sarah and Eva, and the semester at Case Western, were the nurturing environment for my decision to systematically examine the invisible half of the gender-by-late-life interaction.

I elected to take up the project of annotating the literature on older men immediately following the editorial work involved in publishing a collection of original articles about older men's lives. To assure myself of its feasibility I asked three under-graduates to work with me to canvas the available literature in selected areas. This book of annotations directly benefited from the support of those students. Beth E. Hughes, Caren Piela, and Maura A. Kelly helped in spring 1993 to determine the depth of three topics -- retirement, family relations, and health and well-being. Their work went beyond my expectations and is typical of the superb quality colleagues elsewhere find of their better graduate students. In spring 1993 I contracted the volume.

Routinely assisting, reference librarians Alexa Mayo and Tony Stankus were invaluable in tracking down accurate citations to obscurely cited articles, and the staff in the Holy Cross Interlibrary Loan service was a mainstay in keeping the project underway. Thanks to all.

The anticipated hard work of compling an annotated bibliography proved much easier than I ever expected. Finding, reading, and abstracting the 750-plus articles became enjoyable, since I experienced that reward which comes from immersing oneself in a new literature. This result can be shared. This volume in the Gerontology Series adds a new perspective to our familiarity with older men. Thanks to all those researchers "out there" who are sensitive to issues of gender and older men as men.

Introduction

— ♦ —

Studying the gendered lives of elders has become necessary in the study of aging. It is a "gendered" world, and this fact is in evidence across an array of realities. As much as social class, gender directly and indirectly affects longevity and access to societal resources. Gender interacts with age to differentially affect women's and men's late life social relations, self-efficacy and quality of life. Nonetheless, it has been a decade since Alice Rossi (1985) flagged the importance of gender throughout the life course and its near absence in research examining men's and women's late life experiences. Her decade-old observation that gender too often goes unnoted, even though social relations and everyday experiences are structured in important ways along gender lines, still applies to the studies of aging -- social gerontology, geriatric medicine, geropsychiatry, and the psychology of aging. Gender is still too often limited to a census bureau definition, where men and women are mere categories. When gender is recognized as the complex social construction it is, analysis is too frequently limited to the social worlds of older women. The experiences and lives of older men, and the diversity of their experiences, are opaque and hushed by being ignored.

There are reasons for this. One is ageism. Older men are a distinct minority among men, accounting for fifteen percent of the adult male population. Particularly for men, the age structure of society marginalizes and stigmatizes late life. The age structure has divided society since the industrial era into three parts: retirement or leisure for older men, work roles for the middle age, and educational roles for the young (Riley & Riley, 1994). This structural arrangement is *for* middle-aged and younger men and not for older men. It erroneously assumes inevitable declines, and it assumes these declines occur because of aging rather than the self-fulfilling prophecy of a nation's ageism. Older men's pathogenic changes are normalized and taken for granted. Family members and physicians attribute changes in decision-making abilities to normal aging and never consider alternative explanations, such as the side-effects of medications. Even before this, as men approach late life, new, engaging work and work-related opportunities are not offered. Older men are offered golden parachutes and early retirement plans. The spectacle of younger men's work/family juggling draws the audience's attention; men's multiple roles in late life are rarely noticed, even in the new field of men's studies. As these examples suggest, the experiences and lives of older men have been hushed and made invisible.

Among elders, older men are currently outnumbered by older women three to two, and there are just two men for every five women age eighty-five and older. At comparable ages, older women live with more nagging illnesses and frailty than men. As we close this century, women outlive men by an average of seven to eight years, and consequently there are many more frail, unmarried older women noticed in restaurants, churches, and long-term care facilities. For the better part of their late life, many of these women live alone, struggle with the double stigma of being older women, face economic hard times, and eventually become obliged to sell the family home; most face dying without the support of a spouse. These differences in elder sex ratios, longevity, and use of and access to resources have come to mean older men are overbenefited. As a result, their concerns and interests are overlooked as gerontologists redress the struggles of older women.

Until recently, older men were not a social phenomenon commanding great attention. The age structure of society did not seem problematic enough to shift attention away from addressing the masculinities of middle-aged and younger men. Nor did the needs and presence of older men among the elderly provide much of a mandate to examine older men's lives. However, the importance of gender to age, and age to gender, is being acknowledged by both gerontologists and gender scholars. Hendricks (1993) contends that research into aging is sufficiently developed that if we fail to appreciate the importance of gender, we fail to contextualize the aging process. He argues that it is, at this time, egregious to assume all men and all women have comparable experiences despite their gender, social class, and racial/ethnic backgrounds. Thompson (1994) similarly wrote that research into men's lives must appreciate the importance of age -- both chronological age and birth cohort. To make the arrant assumption that masculinity is constructed identically in the culture, in institutions, and in individual's lives across all generations and across a life span is to ignore the significance of age.

The study of gender and aging, and of older men as men, is not unprecedented, just uncommon (cf., Arber & Ginn, 1991; Glasse & Hendricks, 1991; Gutmann, 1987; Thompson, 1994). It is distinct from the vast literature on aged males and the type of information that can be gleaned from this research. It is a smaller body of work which views gender as a relationship, not as an attribute, and consciously brings older men and their lives into the foreground. Much of it is annotated in this volume.

One literature I systematically excluded from annotation is the research which examines effects of aging on physiological, neurological, and cognitive processes. This literature is quite sizable and important itself. But it does not directly speak to men and aging. Rather it examines aging and the sex-specific aging process. For example, in their 1994 Journals of Gerontology article "Influence of letter size on age differences in letter matching" (pp. P24-P28), P. A. Allen, M. B. Patterson, and R. E. Propper examine age differences in information processing. They disregard the gender of the subjects. Much the same, J. B. Aubrey, K. Z. H. Li, and A. R. Dobbs, in a Journals of Gerontology article on "Age differences in the interpretation of misaligned 'you-are-here' maps" (pp. P29-P31), examine the effects of age on a daily activity in a laboratory setting. They observe a sex difference, but do not discuss the finding that men perform faster on contra-aligned maps, although no more accurately than women. These studies do contribute to the fields of gerontology and our understanding of cognitive functioning in late life, and this type of work sometimes attends to sex differences. However, many of these studies still do not even report sex differences. When sex differences are noted, the information provided is about aged males. It is not discussed in terms of older men's v. older women's lives, and gender remains unrecognized.

Another huge body of work not included in this annotation is the clinical and laboratory research on metabolic, hormonal, and biophysiological functioning. This work by physicians and medical scientists often focuses exclusively on older men. The men are studied as an aggregate of human subjects, not as men. G. D. Webb, E. T. Poehlman, and R. P. Tonion, for example, report in their 1993 *Journals of Gerontology* article "Dissociation of changes in metabolic rate and blood pressure with erythrocyte Na-K pump activity in older men after endurance training" (pp. M47-M52) that exercise training increases resting metabolic rate in older men and reduces blood pressure in older, normotensive men, but these changes are dissociated with alterations in the erythrocyte Na-K pump rate. This is an important article on endurance exercise training for healthy older men, and information about older men can be derived from this kind of work. But the authors do not speak directly about men. The piece does not examine gender and aging; instead it was designed to discuss metabolic functioning in older human subjects. Any article like it was thus excluded in this annotation, because what gendered information that can gleaned from the article about older men is only what each reader can extract from it, and gender was not what the authors addressed.

The key inclusion criterion was authors' attention to the interaction of gender and aging. Virtually all articles or chapters included use a comparative framework, and most compare older men to older women. Some compare older men to middle-age and younger men. At times, authors explicitly assess the interaction effect of age by gender; this is most evident in statistical analyses which include the interaction term. At times, the interaction effect is addressed indirectly in the discussion of findings. However approached, the 750-plus articles included in this annotation attend to older men as men, and nearly all were published in the last fifteen years.

A survey of the literature selected for annotation reveals the predominate themes within the studies of older men. Clearly evident is the importance of health and the meaning of work/retirement. Also quite evident is the new place of family relations and the changing nature of other social relationships. What should not be disregarded is the presumption of a distinct masculinity ideology defining late life. An assumption underlying this mushrooming literature on older men is that the "third age" has unique demands, a social script for older men which differs from middle-age and youth. The partitioning of men's lives into three ages appears often. Quite frequently, some form of discontinuity is theorized, for many of the articles abstracted anticipate types of nomic ruptures in men's experiences as they leave middle-age. A smaller number of articles assume that gender governs the gender-by-age interaction, and gender is more a continuous experience across the ages, despite modest age-related changes.

What emerges are ages-of-life models. The assumptions made about discontinuity and continuity are not the same as found in the formal models outlined by Levinson, Erikson, and others. The difference is that these new, commonplace models consciously speak about manhood only, and they do not generalize to the ages-of-life of women. They are more similar to the age-specific masculinities detailed in Rotundo's (1993) historical analysis of the culture of manhood. Thus, the warning flag is up again. We must consider the likelihood that the ages-of-life models that prevail in the research literature only apply to the generation of men currently in late life. These men grew up with World War II, and many with the Depression (Elder, Shanahan, & Clipp, 1994). Unlike what their fathers experienced (Rotundo, 1993) or what their children and grandchildren live with (Goldscheider, 1990; Riley & Riley, 1994), the age structures in society were very pronounced and the prevailing gender ideology defined separate spheres for older men as well. Much of what can be extracted about the gender-by-age interaction from this research literature may well be historically sound yet not generalizable to the next generation of men.

Another unmistakable pattern underlying the annotated literature is the recognition that there are multiple masculinities for older men. There is an appreciation that older men from different classes and racial/ethnic backgrounds do not experience late life uniformly. This awareness of the heterogeneity of older men is an important development, for it has begun to encourage more routine probes into how ethnicity and socioeconomics differentially structure older men's social worlds.

As can be observed by the coverage in this annotated review, some topics related to older men's lives have held greater research attention than others. Older men's religiousness, propensity to take their own life, experiences and special needs in long-term care facilities, sexuality, continued experience of fatherhood, relations with siblings and grandchildren, social relationships after and outside employment, and late life multiple roles have not attracted as much attention and funding as their health experiences and transition to retirement. Many questions remain unaddressed or just partly answered. Even the two heavyweight areas of health and retirement experiences have sizable holes, since early research began with the view that health and retirement are individual experiences, devoid of family attachments, and unconnected to men's adaptations to gender and class ideologies.

Abstracts in the bibliography have been sorted into one of the twelve subject areas. However, virtually all work crosses-over to address issues in areas other than the primary one. These other subject areas are listed in brackets at the end of each abstract, and the numbers conform to chapters and subheadings listed in the table of contents.

References

Arber, S., & Ginn, J. (1991). *Gender and later life: A sociological analysis of resources and constraints*. London: Sage Publications.

Elder, G. H., Shanahan, M. J., & Clipp, E. C. (1994). When war comes to men's lives: Life-course patterns in family, work, and health. *Psychology and Aging, 9*, 5-16.

Glasse, L., & Hendricks, J. (1991). *Gender and aging*. Amityville, NY: Baywood Publishing.

Goldscheider, F. K. (1990). The aging of the gender revolution: What do we know and what do we need to know? *Research on Aging, 12,* 531-545.

Gutmann, D. (1987). *Reclaimed powers: Toward a new psychology of men and women in late life.* New York: Basic Books.

Hendricks, J. (1993). Recognizing the relativity of gender in aging research. *Journal of Aging Studies, 7,* 111-116.

Riley, M. W., & Riley, J. W., Jr. (1994). Age integration and the lives of older people. *The Gerontologist, 34,* 110-115.

Rossi, A. (1985). *Gender and the life course.* New York: Aldine.

Rotundo, E. A. (1993). *American manhood: Transformations in masculinity from the Revolution to the Modern Era.* New York: Basic Books.

Thompson, E. H. (1994). Older men as invisible men in contemporary society. In *Older men's lives* (pp. 1-21). Thousand Oaks, CA: Sage Publications.

MEN
and
AGING

1

Gendered Aging

— ◆ —

IDENTITIES AND AGING

<1>   Barak, B. M., & Stern, B. (1986). Subjective age correlates: A research note. *The Gerontologist, 26,* 571-578.

Reviews the literature and provides an overview of the work examining the age at which individuals perceive themselves as old (or "subjective age"). The authors report that six recent data-based studies indicate no association between subjective age and gender. Earlier writing had suggested that older women would perceive themselves as younger than men in their age-cohort, but this difference is not evident. [1.1, 6.2]

<2>   Cremin, M. C. (1992). Feeling old versus being old: Views of troubled aging. *Social Science and Medicine, 34,* 1305-1315.

Describes the experiences of aging constructed by five older people, their adult children, and a team of health professionals evaluating their health status. Older participants, who range in age from 69 to 86, make a clear distinction between being old and feeling old; their children did not. No elder identifies self as old although each recalls specific and transient episodes of feeling old. Their children see the parent as being old; and their understanding is that their parents are in a process of inevitable and irreversible decline. The involvement of the clinic generates yet another construction. The study explores the impact these sometimes conflicting views have. The phenomenon of troubled aging is seen as a feature of the children's experience of their parents' aging, not as a central aspect of the older people's experience. [1.1, 6.2]

<3>   Fultz, N. H., & Herzog, A. R. (1991). Gender differences in affiliation and instrumentality across adulthood. *Psychology and Aging, 6,* 579-586.

Observes the renewed interest in age-related gender differences, particularly regarding the possibility that men and women become more similar in older age. Tests the hypothesis that gender differences decline across adulthood. Data are from the 1971 Quality of American Life and 1976 Americans View Their Mental Health surveys; six measures of dimensions of affiliation and instrumentality are assessed. For each measure, the variance explained by age, gender, and the age X gender interaction term is compared with the variance explained by age and gender alone. The interaction term did not increase the explained variance for any measure, which argues against a late-life convergence perspective. Since release from active parenting is proposed as a basis for gender convergence, re-examining the data by limiting the analyses to respondents with children does not change the conclusion. [1.1, 1.3]

<4>   Goldsmith, R. E., & Heiens, R. A. (1992). Subjective age: A test of five hypotheses. *The Gerontologist, 32*, 312-317.

Subjective age, or how old a person perceives self to be, is thought to be an important perspective for the aging process. Addresses five age-related hypotheses based on subjective aging for 607 adults. Finds that subjective age is not as close in agreement with chronological age as are ratings of feeling one's age and looking one's age. Men and women do not differ on these two dimensions of the experience of aging. Suggests that researchers simply neglect to focus on the appearance aspect of men's lives, and it seems men feel the same pressures to be young as women. [1.1]

<5>   Gradman, T. J. (1989). *Does work make the man?: A review of research on retirement.* Santa Monica, CA: Rand Corporation.

This report reviews the literature on the relationships among retirement, masculine identity, and work identity. The close relationship between masculine identity and work identity has rarely been studied empirically, especially among older men. The closest studies to this area have shown that identification with work is negatively correlated with positive retirement attitudes and a good adjustment to retirement. Some studies have begun to look at how men's gender-role and values change throughout the lifespan, particularly in later years. The overall finding suggests some lessening of the importance of previous male-female differences. [1.1, 10.2]

<6>   Gradman, T. J. (1994). Masculine identity from work to retirement. In E. Thompson (Ed.), *Older men's lives* (pp. 104-121). Thousand Oaks, CA: Sage Publications.

Probes late-life masculine identity as men experience the transition to retirement. Theorizes that older men's gender identity evolves as they age; they confront continuous traditional masculinity expectations as well as a gradual press for more affiliation-oriented feminine behavior. Examining work identification and masculine identity at different stages of retirement reveals gender identity fluctuates throughout the transition, and finds setting the date of retirement marks a greater threat to identity and well-being than being retired. Concludes that it is the perceived loss of the masculine turf of the workplace, not the experience of being retired, which affects psychological continuity. [1.1, 10.2]

<7>   Gray, H., & Dressel, P. (1985). Alternative interpretations of aging among gay males. *The Gerontologist, 25*, 83-87.

Investigates prevailing myths and stereotypes about aging homosexuals (e.g., growing older and being unable to find a partner because of the stigma of aging) using data from 4,212 gay men. The diversity among aging gay men is studied by controlling for the length of time engaged in homosexual activity. Similar to heterosexuals, older gay men are likely to experience declining positive feelings about their age and appearance. Among gays, subcultural opportunities and length of subcultural socialization affect openness about one's lifestyle. The findings suggest there are cohort effects -- e.g., the oldest gay men, who grew up in historical periods that were intolerant of homosexuality, prefer less openness. [1.1, 6.1]

<8>   Harris, M. B. (1994). Growing old gracefully: Age concealment and gender. *Journals of Gerontology: Psychological Sciences, 49*, P149-P158.

Investigates some of the relationships between age concealment and gender with questionnaire data from 269 adults age 18-80. Finds that most of the signs of aging are considered unattractive for both males and females, but aging men are not judged as severely as aging women. Men are less likely to use age concealment techniques, and elders who conceal their age are judged more harshly. These findings are consistent with two different double standards of aging--one indicating that aging is judged differently depending on gender, and one indicating the people judge use of age concealment more harshly in others than self. [1.1]

<9>   Hubley, A. M., & Hultsch, D. F. (1994). The relationship of personality trait variables to subjective age identity in older adults. *Research on Aging, 16*, 415-439.

Examines the relationship between personality trait characteristics and subjective age identity with two elderly samples. Asked 241 community-dwelling adults age 55-75 and 355 adults age 55-85 the age they feel (felt age) and the age they would like to be (ideal age). Finds internal locus of control and extraversion are related to felt age; powerful-other locus of control, neuroticism, extraversion and openness to experience are related to ideal age. Correlations between felt and ideal age are low and positive in both samples. No meaningful age by gender interactions are observed. [1.1]

<10>   Hyde, J. S., & Phillis, D. E. (1979). Androgyny across the life span. *Developmental Psychology, 15*, 334-336.

A survey of 289 people age 13-85 indicates that men become more androgynous with age and women less so. These interpretations are not based on continuous scoring of the Bem Sex-Role Inventory. Rather, categorical scoring, which classifies each individual as either feminine, masculine, androgynous, or undifferentiated, indicates a rise in androgyny among men as age increases and a concomitant decline among women. The increase among older men is predicted, but the decrease among older women runs counter to expectation. Concludes older women may have difficulty rating themselves on such traits as "athletic" and "ambitious," and the Bem Sex Role Inventory may have youthful masculine traits but no masculine traits which would apply throughout the life span. [1.1, 1.3]

<11>   Jacobs, R. H. (1994). His and her aging: Differences, difficulties, dilemmas, delights. *Journal of Geriatric Psychiatry, 27*, 113-128.

Summarizes gender-specific issues of aging, and outlines strategies for helping both men and women deal with the differences, difficulties, dilemmas, and delights of aging. Discusses ten areas in which people can choose how they age, including accepting aging, acknowledging rage, taking care of self, and growing and changing. Suggestions for men include lessening dependence on wives for companionship, lessening alcohol use, making social contacts, and participating in community and other activities. Therapeutic intervention needs to focus on helping older men find ways to replace lost status, activities, and contacts. Concludes noting that men and women share more in common on that journey than their differences. [1.1, 7.1, 12.3]

<12>   Janelli, L. M. (1993). Are there body image differences between older men and women? *Western Journal of Nursing Research, 15*, 327-339.

Studies the relationship between gender and body image among 39 men age 63-93 and 50 women age 60-98 who reside in long-term care facilities. Finds no indication that men are more or less dissatisfied than women with their body as measured by the Body-Cathexis scale, but men are more dissatisfied with aspects of self. These findings support the premise that gender and cultural values regarding aging influence how older men view men's and their own bodies. [1.1]

<13>   Kivett, V. R. (1991). Centrality of the grandfather role among older rural black and white men. *Journals of Gerontology: Social Sciences, 46*, S250-S258.

Examines racial differences in the centrality of the grandfather role and factors related to its saliency. Although black and white men rank the importance of the grandfather role similarly, the identity is more central to older black men. Interaction between the grandchild and grandfather is affected by blacks' fluid family boundaries, affection for grandchildren, exchanges of help, and racial differences in norms of noninterference, intergenerational involvement and association with the grandchildren. Discusses the evidence for cultural distinctions underlying the grandfather role. [1.1, 8.3]

<14>   McCreary, D. R. (1990). Self-perceptions of life-span gender-role develop-ment. *International Journal of Aging and Human Development, 31*, 135-146.

Debates whether masculine and feminine gender-role attributes remain stable across the life-span. Reports two studies in which participants assess their own life-span gender role variability based upon their past and expected future performance in age-related developmental tasks. In one study, college undergraduates rate themselves at the present time and in two prospective points--parenthood and retirement--on their gender attributes. In the next, elders rated themselves at the present time and in two retrospective points--work-entry and parenthood. Attributes vary significantly as a result of the "developmental period," and are rated least like self at the earlier period (work-entry). Both masculinity and femininity increase from that marker period. [1.1, 1.5]

<15>   Myers, W. A. (1989). I can't play ball anymore. *Journal of Geriatric Psychiatry, 22*, 121-139.

Presents four case vignettes of elderly men age 69-74 with late-life depressions precipitated by physical illness and disability. The illness and disability result in the final loss of ability to perform long-standing athletic activities. Discusses how athletic skills are developed in the context of an earlier self, and how the loss of the athletic function led to a double loss involving aspects of self and ties to important objects. [1.1]

<16> Ogilvie, D. M. (1987). **Life satisfaction and identity structure in late middle-aged men and women.** *Psychology and Aging, 2,* 217-224.

Studies the situated identities of 17 retirement-age men and 15 women to determine the amount of time spent in each identity and the importance of each to life-satisfaction. Observes no gender differences, and finds support the hypothesis that satisfaction-with-life is a function of the amount of time an individual spends in major identities as well as with health status. The research shows the important of enacting major identities in later life (e.g., grandfather v. stamp collector), and how they give individuals access to full self-expression and meaning in life. [1.1, 2.3]

<17> Puglisi, J. T. (1983). **Self-perceived age changes in sex role self concept.** *International Journal of Aging and Human Development, 16,* 183-191.

Uses the Bem Sex Role Inventory to assess gender identity in 62 students, their middle-aged and elderly family members. All three generations rate themselves retrospectively and/or prospectively, describing themselves at age 20, at age 45, and at age 70. Results do not support the hypothesis that men and women experience convergence in gender identity in later life. Rather, parallel patterns of development emerge for men and women. In all three ages men and women report high masculine self-descriptions to middle age, followed by decreases in masculinity in later life. [1.1, 1.3]

<18> Puglisi, J. T., & Jackson, D. W. (1980-81). **Self role identity and self esteem in adulthood.** *International Journal of Aging and Human Development, 12,* 129-138.

Examines sex role orientation and self esteem in a sample of 2,069 Ohio State University students, employees, and alumni age 17 to 81. Finds no support for the hypothesis of a convergence of gender in later life. Rather, men and women evidence parallel patterns of gender identification across the age range studied. Men and women display peak masculinity in the middle years, men reveal a curvilinear pattern with masculinity peaking in their forties, and no differences in femininity scores are noted. Masculinity is a better predictor of self esteem than femininity. [1.1, 1.5]

<19> Rakowski, W., & Hickey, T. (1992). **Mortality and the attribution of health problems to aging among older adults.** *American Journal of Public Health, 82,* 1139-1141.

Determines the association between mortality and self-attributions of health problems to aging. Data are on 1,391 respondents from the Longitudinal Study of Aging who have difficulty with activities in daily living. From the sample, 72 persons attribute impairment primarily to "old age." Logistic regression analyses showed these attributions increased the risk of mortality 1.78 times. Concludes that attributing health problems to aging may very well carry a risk of adverse health events. [1.1, 2.1]

<20> **Rubinstein, R. L. (1986).** *Singular paths: Old men living alone.* **New York: Columbia University Press.**

Based on interviews with older men living on their own, some who are "isolates" and some who were regular attendees at a senior center, the book provides an important review of the lives of this population of older men--their activities, social relations, loneliness, sense of place in a neighborhood, experience with widowhood, and identity as men living alone. [2.1, 7.5]

<21> **Ryff, C. D. (1991). Possible selves in adulthood and old age: A tale of shifting horizons.** *Psychology and Aging, 6,* **286-295.**

Determines how adults conceive of their personal progress or decline over the course of adult life. Data are on how young, middle-aged and elderly adults (N = 308) evaluate their present, past, future, and ideal self-assessments on six dimensions of psychological well-being. Older men recall past levels of personal growth significantly higher than present ratings. Recollections of the past-to-present trajectory indicate a perception of similar or stable levels of functioning in some domains (autonomy, positive relations with others, environmental mastery for men, purpose in life for women), progress in other domains (self acceptance for both men and women, environmental mastery and positive relations with others for women) and declines in other realms (purpose in life and personal growth for men). [1.1, 1.3, 2.4]

<22> **Seccombe, K., & Ishii-Kuntz, M. (1991). Perceptions of problems associated with aging: Comparisons among four older age cohorts.** *The Gerontologist, 31,* **527-533.**

With data on 2,329 noninstitutionalized adults, addresses how the elderly perceive the aging process. Examines the perceptions of aging and concern over special problems faced by the elderly among four age cohorts: the middle-aged (55-64), the young-old (65-74), the old (75-84), and the oldest-old (85+). Men are described as becoming "old" between 60-64 and women are "old" several years earlier, between 55-59. The middle-aged cohort is the most pessimistic, envisioning more problems associated with aging. Despite greater experience with functional and social difficulties, the oldest old are surprisingly optimistic in their view of aging. Concludes the perceptions by the oldest old cohort are more likely than other elders' attitudes to depend on this group's assessment of their own personal problems. [1.1, 2.4]

<23> **Solomon, K., & Szwabo, P. A. (1994). The work-oriented culture: Success and power in elderly men. In E. Thompson (Ed.),** *Older men's lives* **(pp. 42-64). Thousand Oaks, CA: Sage Publications.**

Addresses how the meanings of work, power, success, and self are integrated by the traditional masculinity ideology, which guides the experiences of one cohort of older men--those born between the end of the Victorian era and the onset of the Great Depression. Theorizes that external experiences change the outward behaviors of many of these men, but their self-concept is consistent with the gender ideology they integrated early in life. Expressions of their masculinity are still found in unpaid and paid work or work-related activity. Concludes that men face many developmental stresses as they strive to maintain the gendered self. [1.1, 1.5]

<24> Thomas, L. E., Kraus, P. A., & Chambers, K. O. (1990). Metaphoric analysis of meaning in the lives of elderly men: A cross-cultural investigation. *Journal of Aging Studies, 4*, 1-15.

This article reports on the nuances of imagination and belief which lie behind the ways elders communicate the meaning and purpose of their lives. Explicit and implicit metaphors are analyzed as a means of determining personal meaning in the lives of 70 elderly English and Indian men. Analysis of the metaphors indicate marked differences in their psychological worlds, with English men more privatized and stoic and the Indian men expressing strong achievement concerns. [1.1]

LIFE REVIEW

<25> David, D. (1990). Reminiscence, adaptation, and social context in old age. *International Aging and Human Development, 30*, 175-188.

Theorizes that reminiscence is adaptive in late life. Research has not yet produced consistent findings to support theory, perhaps because researchers have not considered social context or the content of reminiscing. In an exploratory study of residents in two retirement communities, observes strikingly different patterns of reminiscing and well-being. For widowed men, elaboration of memories, life reviewing, and high importance of others are associated with positive adaptation (life satisfaction and self-esteem). [1.2, 2.3]

<26> DeGenova, M. K. (1992). If you had your life to live over again: What would you do differently? *International Journal of Aging and Human Development, 34*, 135-143.

Argues that life review is a natural process occurring in later life. Identifies what 122 retired elderly persons would do differently if they had their lives to live over again. Based on a questionnaire assessing life revision in areas of friends, family, work, education, religion, leisure, and health, the greatest amount of desired change is the area of education. Men would spend more time pursuing their education, and women would spend time developing their mind or intellect. When controlled for health, social activity, and income, educational level is the most significant predictor of life revision. Concludes that both attained and longed-for education are highly valued. [1.2]

<27> Rybarczyk, B. D., & Auerbach, S. M. (1990). Reminiscence interviews as stress management interventions for older patients undergoing surgery. *The Gerontologist, 30*, 522-527.

Evaluates the efficacy of reminiscence interviews as a stress management intervention for elder persons facing major surgery. Age-peer interviews with 104 elderly men do not elicit significantly greater overall reductions in state anxiety or increases in coping self-efficacy scores than nonpeers, but do produce significantly higher coping self-efficacy scores than nonpeers when administering a challenge reminiscence interview. [1.2, 2.3]

<28> Wong, P. T., & Watt, L. M. (1991). What types of reminiscence are associated with successful aging? *Psychology and Aging, 6*, 272-279.

Examines the controversy regarding the adaptive benefits of reminiscence, and investigates what types of reminiscence are associated with successful aging for 88 men and women judged to be aging successfully and 83 men and women aging unsuccessfully. Successful aging is operationally defined as higher than average ratings in mental and physical health and adjustment. All elders are 65 to 95, and approximately half living in the community and half in institutions. On the basis of prior research, six types of reminiscence were identified: integrative, instrumental, transmissive, narrative, escapist, and obsessive. As predicted, successful agers showed significantly more integrative and instrumental reminiscence but less obsessive reminiscence than their unsuccessful counterparts. Community dwellers also showed more instrumental and integrative reminiscence than institutionalized seniors showed. [1.2, 2.2]

MEN'S LATER LIFE PERSONALITY

<29>   Bar-Yam, M. (1991). Do women and men speak in different voices? A comparative study of self-evolvement. *International Journal of Aging and Human Development, 32*, 247-259.

Because most developmental theories use men's development as the norm and women's development as a deviation, compares women's and men's levels of self evolvement, as defined by Kegan's constructive-developmental theory. Finds no sex difference in evolvement, and no support for men's "advantage" or women's "different voice." Although the difference is not statistically significant, finds men are more often than women in earlier developmental stages involving embeddedness in relationships (rather than autonomy). Instructive are the ways people express themselves, describe their experiences, and make meaning of their life and social reality. Many men's statements are contrary to stereotype and focus on a "care ethic" -- defining themselves as nurturing and emotionally attached. Concludes that yearning for inclusion and separateness may not be gendered, rather salient for both older men and women. [1.3, 1.5]

<30>   Barer, B. M. (1994). Men and women aging differently. *International Journal of Aging and Human Development, 38*, 29-40.

Explores the implications of gender differences in health, SES, and social resources that persist into advanced old age and result in variations in life trajectories and responses to the challenge of longevity. Uses a sample of 39 community-dwelling white men and 111 women age 85 and older from the San Francisco 85+ Study. Finds the majority of the women are unmarried, lived alone, and have activity restrictions. Men have fewer problems with functional limitations, maintain a higher level of activity--being more involved in hobbies, household maintenance, and organizations--and exercise more independence. An analysis of gender variations in life trajectories, however, illustrates some disadvantages for the men: Their well-being can be undermined by unanticipated events such as widowhood, caregiving, and relocation. Women experience widowhood at a younger age, giving them time to adjust to their loss and greater continuity in their late-life activities and relationships. [1.3, 1.4]

<31>   Barrick, A. L., Hutchinson, R. L., & Deckers, L. H. (1990). Humor, aggression and aging. *The Gerontologist, 30*, 675-678.

Observes that humor as an emotion has rarely been studied in elders. Investigates humor response and arousal to aggressive cartoons among 154 young and elderly men and women. People rated the degree of pain suffered by cartoon characters and the funniness of cartoons. Finds gender differences, but no effects for age. Men rate cartoons funnier than women, and for men, there is no relationship between perceived pain and funniness. [1.3]

<32> **Belsky, J. (1992). The research findings on gender issues in aging men and women. In B. R. Wainrib (Ed.), *Gender issues across the life cycle* (pp. 163-171). New York: Springer.**

Emphasizes the remarkable resilience of an almost-40-year-old finding about gender and later life, and just how difficult it really is to say that men and women shed or even mute their masculine and feminine identities in their later years. Contends that people may indeed become somewhat freer in general to express their assertive or nurturing tendencies in the second half of adult life, but basic predispositions, values, expectations, and ways of reacting to the world seem just as firmly determined by gender in old age as they are in younger years. [1.3, 1.5]

<33> **Butcher, J. N., Aldwin, C. M., Levenson, M. R., Ben-Porath, Y. S., Spiro, A. 3d., & Bosse, R. (1991). Personality and aging: A study of the MMPI-2 among older men. *Psychology & Aging*, 6, 361-370.**

Questions whether separate norms for older men are necessary for the revised Minnesota Multiphasic Personality Inventory (MMPI-2). Scores from 1,459 men in the Normative Aging Study are contrasted with those from younger and middle-aged men from the MMPI Restandardization Study. There are few differences between the two groups. Concludes that special, age-related norms for the MMPI-2 are not needed for older men. [1.3]

<34> **Carmelli, D., Dame, A., & Swan, G. E. (1992). Age-related changes in behavioral components in relation to changes in global Type A behavior. *Journal of Behavioral Medicine*, 15, 143-154.**

Investigates long-term changes of the Type A behavior pattern in 565 men age 65-86 who participated in an earlier (1964) study. Test-retest correlations for seven behavioral components of the structured interview support the premise of moderate stability in personality. Significant mean changes are observed for Type A content, exactingness, competitiveness, and hostility. Also, changes in competitiveness and hostility are Type A dependent. [1.3]

<35> **Chowdhary, U. (1990). Notion of control and self-esteem of institutionalized older men. *Perceptual & Motor Skills*, 70, 731-738.**

Assesses the influence of control on the self-esteem (feelings of self-worth) for institutionalized elderly men (N = 12). Analysis indicate that having input in decision-making process can enhance institutionalized elderly men's self-esteem and contribute toward improving their quality of life. [1.3, 11.1]

<36>   Costa, P. T. Jr., & McCrae, R. R. (1988). Personality in adulthood: A six-
       year longitudinal study of self-reports and spouse ratings on the NEO
       Personality Inventory. *Journal of Personality and Social Psychology, 54,*
       853-863.

Gathers self-reports (N = 983) and spouse ratings (N = 167) on the NEO Personality
Inventory, which measures five dimensions of normal personality. Finds in these data
from men and women age 21-96 evidence of small declines in activity, positive
emotions, and openness to actions which might be attributed to maturation. However, in
longitudinal analyses none of these effects was replicated. Retest stability is quite high
for all five dimensions in self-reports and for the three dimensions measured at both
times in spouse ratings. Concludes that personality is stable after age 30. [1.3]

<37>   Costa, P. T. Jr., Metter, E. J., & McCrae, R. R. (1994). Personality stability
       and its contribution to successful aging. *Journal of Geriatric Psychiatry,*
       27, 41-59.

Discusses how the stability of personality contributes to successful aging. Personality
traits are basic tendencies that, with external influences such as family history and job
training, affect adaptation, the self-concept, and biography. Argues that personality
dispositions provide a dependable basis for adaptation to a changing world -- declining
health, economic hardships, death of a loved one, or retirement -- through the use of
skills and styles developed over a lifetime. Several longitudinal studies offer remarkably
similar conclusions: Personality is largely stable in adulthood, even in the face of
serious medical conditions. Concludes that personal traits form a central part of how
people view themselves, and the continued sense that we remain the same person
depends in part on having the same social, emotional, and motivational styles over long
periods of time. We are what we are--and the recognition of that fact is a crucial step in
successful aging. [1.3, 2.2]

<38>   Croake, J. W., Myers, K. M., & Singh, A. (1988). The fears expressed by
       elderly men and women: A lifespan approach. *International Journal of*
       Aging and Human Development, 26, 139-146.

Comments how little work has examined adult fears, specifically in an elderly population.
Finds that older men express less fearfulness than older women, which is a gender
difference one observes in children and adolescents. When compared to other adult
groups, there are differences on several categories of fears. The elderly group rank
aging and sickness as their foremost fears. Results suggest that some fears may
change or intensify over the lifespan, and within each period men report less fearfulness
than women. [1.3]

<39>   Dean-Church, L., & Gilroy, F. D. (1993). Relation of sex-role orientation to
       life satisfaction in a healthy elderly sample. *Journal of Social Behavior and*
       Personality, 8, 133-140.

Examines whether gender outlook (i.e., gender orientation) is predictive of life
satisfaction in a sample noninstitutionalized 50 older men and 50 older women age 55-
92. The study also assesses the role of masculinity and femininity in promoting life
satisfaction. Finds an androgynous orientation (i.e., high scores on both masculine and

feminine dimensions) is associated with greater life satisfaction in the active elderly. Older men with a traditional masculine sex-typed orientation fall below, but not significantly below androgynous men and have life satisfaction scores almost identical to traditionally feminine women. Thus, although stereotypically feminine or expressive characteristics are not particularly adaptive for young men, they may serve the population of older men. [1.3, 2.3]

<40> Degelman, D., Owens, S. A., Reynolds, T., & Riggs, J. (1991). Age and gender differences in beliefs about personal power and injustice. *International Journal of Aging and Human Development, 33,* 101-111.

Explores belief in a just world as it relates to the demographic factors of age and gender. College students and community-dwelling adults age 60-86 are compared on attitude scales assessing personal power and belief that conditions can be unjust. Finds one age by gender interaction--older men do not differ from younger men and women on personal power, rather it was older women who report much lower personal power scores. Both older and younger men are predictably less likely than women to believe that conditions in the world can be unjust, and this belief does not differ as a function of age. [1.3]

<41> de Vries, B., Bluck, S., & Birren, J. E. (1993). The understanding of death and dying in a life-span perspective. *The Gerontologist, 33,* 366-372.

Reviews how prior work on attitudes toward death generally finds age and gender effects, such that elders are less frightened by and more likely to talk and think about death than other age groups, and men are less anxious about death than women. Codes the content of essays about death and dying written by fifty-four men and women of different ages. No gender difference or gender by age interaction is found. Rather, for both men and women, discussions of death are more frequent and more complex than discussions of dying, reveal low levels of acceptance, and refer to others more often than to self. [1.3, 2.3, 2.5]

<42> Erber, J. T., Szuchman, L. T., & Rothberg, S. T. (1990). Age, gender, and individual differences in memory failure appraisal. *Psychology and Aging, 5,* 600-603.

Examines how age and gender affect appraisal of others. Young adults (22 men and 24 women) and older adults (24 men and 24 women) rated 12 gender-neutral vignettes describing short-, long-, and very-long-term memory failure. Target persons were young or older men or women. Participants from both gender and age groups use a double standard. Failures of older targets of both genders are rated as signifying greater mental difficulty. [1.3, 6.1]

<43> Feifel, H., & Strack, S. (1987). Old is old is old? *Psychology and Aging, 2,* 409-412.

Analyzes Neugrarten's premise of within-group heterogeneity among elders. Compares matched samples of white, healthy elderly men who are young-old (age 65-74) and old-old (age 75 and older). Although statistically significant differences are sometimes present, the pattern of no differences is more common. Broad similarities characterize the two ages. No differences are manifest in areas as fear of death, religious belief, life values, general mood, self-concept, and perceived social support. [1.3, 6.2]

<44> Field, D., & Millsap, R. E. (1991). Personality in advanced old age: Continuity or change? *Journals of Gerontology: Psychological Sciences,* *46,* **P299-P308.**

Long-term continuity of personality has remained an uncertainty and required waiting for longitudinal studies. Studying the survivors among the Berkeley Older Generation Study, considerable continuity is found for four of the "big five" traits between 1969 and 1983. Change is also apparent. Men report higher satisfaction than women, and this difference is stable over time. For the intellect component, there is a gender-by-time interaction--men's advantage in rate of intellect declines vasnishes. Overtime there also is an increase in agreeableness and a decline in extroversion. [1.3]

<45> Giambra, L., Camp, C. J., & Grodsky, A. (1992). Curiosity and stimulation seeking across the adult life span: Cross-sectional and 6- to 8-year longitudinal findings. *Psychology and Aging, 7,* **150-157.**

Earlier studies show information-seeking (i.e., curiosity) does not systematically change across the adult life span, but stimulation-seeking (i.e., boredom and need for external stimulation) significantly decreases with age. Replicates these outcomes using cross-sectional samples of 1,356 men and 1,080 women age 17-92, and longitudinal information 6-8 years afterward on 222 men and 124 women. Because information seeking seems unabated by aging, men's curiosity is not related to aging. Finds significant declines for simulation seeking until late adulthood. Proposes explanations for why senescence people are less bored and in less need for external stimulation. [1.3]

<46> Gray, A., Jackson, D. N., & McKinlay, J. B. (1991). The relation between dominance, anger, and hormones in normally aging men: Results from the Massachusetts Male Aging Study. *Psychosomatic Medicine, 53,* **375-385.**

Examines the relation of two personality characteristics (dominance and anger) to hormones in normally aging men. Comparing the Personality Research Form Dominance subscale and the Spielberger Anger Expression scale to serum levels of 17 endocrine variables, including testosterone (T), dihydrotestosterone, cortisol, and prolactin in 1,709 men age 39 to 70, finds a dominant personality profile with some aggressive behavior related to weaker androgens, biologically active T, and T that can rapidly dissociate from the albumin to enter tissues. Results partially support a relationship between T and aggression and/or dominance. [1.3]

<47> Gutmann, D., & Huyck, M. H. (1994). Development and pathology in postparental men: A community study. In E. Thompson (Ed.), *Older men's lives* **(pp. 65-84). Thousand Oaks, CA: Sage Publications.**

Extends the theory that older men experience reorganization of their psychosexual nature in the transition to postparental life, and proposes that for some men, the strains of adapting to the masculinity associated with postparental life result in psychopathology. Victims of late-onset psychopathology, these men react negatively to the new developmental tides. Data on 107 men in Huyck's Parkville sample affirm a typology identifying which men are most vulnerable to late-onset distress. Those who manifest late-onset pathogenesis react to late life demands for androgyny and unresolved early life developmental failures. Unlike irreversible losses, disorders of developmental origin are reversible and treatable. [1.3, 1.5]

<48> Hess, T. M., Vandermaas, M. O., Donley, J., & Snyder, S. S. (1987). **Memory for sex-role consistent and inconsistent actions in young and old adults.** *Journal of Gerontology, 42,* 505-511.

Studies schematic influences on memory retention in adulthood and searches for age differences in the flexibility of schematic processing. In the first experimental protocol, young and older men read statements describing a man performing actions consistent or inconsistent with his prescribed gender role. Although older men's own gender-role orientation is more traditional, both age groups attribute more masculine traits to the traditional target. Observed in both experiments, people alter their processing of information relative to the gender role emphasized for the target; the schematic effect is stronger for men than women. No age effects on flexibility are observed. [1.3, 6.2]

<49> Howard, J. H., Rechnitzer, P. A., Cunningham, D. A., & Donner, A. P. (1986). **Change in Type A behavior a year after retirement.** *The Gerontologist, 26,* 643-649.

Data from a one-year prospective study of 224 men indicate that the magnitude of Type A behavior changes in the Type B direction after one year of normal retirement. Randomized to a control group or an exercise group (which met 2-3 times weekly and replicates a work-activity group), findings show the men in the control group (who represent "normal" retirement), who were blue collar workers, and whose fitness improved move in the Type B direction. Type A men show improvements in mental health, and improvements in cardiovascular fitness reduces their Type A behavior, particularly the hostility component. [1.3, 10.2]

<50> Huyck, M. H. (1991). **Predicates of personal control among middle-aged and young-old men and women in middle America.** *International Journal of Aging and Human Development, 32,* 261-275.

Some evidence indicates a sense of control is particularly important in maintaining well-being in late life. Theorizes contemporary American men shift patterns of personal investment from the emphasis on paid work in middle age to considering retirement. Finds no gender difference in the sense of control, satisfaction with life domains, or psychological investment in these domains, but gender predicts which life domains afford a sense of control. For older men, satisfaction with work, lower psychological investment in work and greater investment in marriage contribute to a sense of control. Findings are consistent with Gutmann's model of men's development. [1.3, 1.5]

<51> Kunen, S., Tang, W., & Overstreet, S. (1992). **Older adults' judgments of historically important events: The roles of gender, age, and education.** *Educational Gerontology, 18,* 193-212.

Asks middle-age and elderly individuals to list the 10 most important events that have happened in the United States since 1900, and these lists are analyzed as a function of gender, age, and education. Few gender differences in value judgments are obtain, which provides mixed support for the notion that gender and age are related in systematic ways to value judgments. Findings are discussed in the context of Gilligan's theory of gender differences in values, and Erikson's and Gutmann's theories of age-related gender changes in values. [1.3, 1.5]

<52> Labouvie-Vief, G., DeVoe, M., & Bulka, D. (1989). Speaking about feelings: Conceptions of emotion across the life span. *Psychology and Aging, 4,* 425-437.

Defines adulthood as developmental movements which have significant implications for the ways in which individuals regulate their thinking and action. Addresses one area of self-regulation--how individuals conceptualize their emotional processes. Self-descriptions of emotions (anger, sadness, fear, and happiness) by 72 participants age 10-77 are scored for developmental complexity. Younger people describe emotions in terms of sensorimotor actions, outer appearance, and an emphasis on control and the ideal. Older participants convey a vivid sense of emotional experience and bodily sensations. Men are as likely to convey emotions in a mature manner, but they are also more likely to endorse coping and defense strategies which involved turning against the self and could mute development and emotional experience. [1.1, 1.3, 1.5]

<53> Labouvie-Vief, G., Hakim-Larson, J., & Hobart, C. J. (1987). Age, ego level, and life-span development of coping and defense processes. *Psychology and Aging, 2,* 286-293.

Examines coping and defense strategy use in a sample of 100 men and women age 10-77. Finds that, in addition to age, the developmental measures of ego level and source of stress predict the use of particular coping and defense strategies. Concludes that there is a need to go beyond the distinction between problem-focused and emotion-focused coping to specify developmental variations of less and more mature levels. Similarly, the stylistic gender differences which reveal men less likely than women to avoid confrontations, accept personal blame for stressful encounters and rely on social support networks to cope may be measurement instrument artifacts, for measures cannot reveal the range of actual strategies individuals use. [1.3, 1.5]

<54> Lee, G. R., & Shehan, C. L. (1989). Social relations and self-esteem of older persons. *Research on Aging, 11,* 427-442.

Examines the antecedents of self-esteem among elders. Theoretically, central to self-esteem is the ability of the individual to terminate personal relations (e.g., friendships v. kin relations) that could yield negative appraisals. Consistent with premise, friendship interaction is positively related to self-esteem, whereas kinship interaction is not. Among men, this relationship is stronger among the retired than the employed. Marital satisfaction also affects self-esteem positively, more so for retired men. [1.3, 8.4, 7.3]

<55> Levenson, R. W., Carstensen, L. L., Friesen, W. V., & Ekman, P. (1991). Emotion, physiology, and expression in old age. *Psychology and Aging, 6,*

28-35.

Old age provides a unique opportunity to study emotion at the end point of what might be a lifelong process of emotional development. Examines emotion-specific autonomic nervous system activity in 20 elders. Among the findings are that elderly men and women do not differ in emotional physiology or facial expression, and elderly men report experiencing less intense emotions when reliving emotional memories than elderly women. Discusses how this latter finding raises interesting questions about how men experience emotional experiences initially and at recall. [1,1, 1.3]

<56> Malatesta-Magai, C., Jonas, R., Shepart, B., & Culver, L. C. (1992). Type A behavior pattern and emotion expression in young and older adults. *Psychology and Aging, 7*, 551-561.

Suggests that research on personality effects on illness and aging "came of age" over the past two decades. Compares the relationships found between Type A behavior and anxiety, depression, anger, aggression, hostility, and anger-in-anger-out. Data are from 80 younger (average age = 28) and 80 older (average age = 69) men and women. The greater expressivity among the elders challenges earlier claims that the emotionality of older individuals declines with age and becomes more blunted. Expected and finds men less emotion-masking than women and less conflicted about the expression of anger. [1.3]

<57> McCrae, R. R., Costa, P. T. Jr., & Arenberg, D. (1980). Constancy of adult personality structure in males: Longitudinal, cross-sectional, and times-of-measurement analysis. *Journal of Gerontology, 35*, 877-883.

Questions whether personality is stable in adulthood, and compares the factor structure of temperament scales longitudinally in three administrations six years apart and cross-sectionally in three age cohorts. Men (N = 769) from the Baltimore Longitudinal Study of Aging were age 17-92 at the time of the first administration. Finds no systematic evidence of variation in structure across groups. This invariance of personality structure suggests the stability of personality organization throughout the adults years. [1.3]

<58> Mroczek, D. K., Spiro, A. 3d., Aldwin, C. M., Ozer, D. J., & Bosse, R. (1993). Construct validation of optimism and pessimism in older men: Findings from the normative aging study. *Health Psychology, 12*, 406-409.

Suggests that the constructs of optimism and pessimism may be not bipolar, but separate constructs and indistinguishable from other personality traits in older men, such as neuroticism and extroversion. Examines the associations of separate optimism and pessimism measures with self-reports of hassles, psychological symptoms, and illness severity, controlling for personality among the 1,192 men from the Normative Aging Study. The findings suggest optimism and pessimism are separate; although attenuated, their relation to external criteria remain when controlled. [1.3]

<59> Pitcher, B. L., Spykerman, B. R., & Gazi-Tabatabaie, M. (1987). Stability of perceived personal control for older black and while men. *Research on Aging, 9*, 200-225.

The life-span perspective increases attention to the issue of stability versus change in adult personality and behavior. Data on men from the National Longitudinal Survey are used to investigate perceived personal control over time. Finds the meaning of personal control is not equivalent between black and white men. Over the course of seven years, the structure of personal control remains stable for each group. Black men's level of control (more external) remained stable over the three panels, but whites show some evidence of becoming more external with age. [1.3]

<60> Plouffe, L., & Gravelle F. (1989). Age, sex, and personality correlates of self-actualization in elderly adults. *Psychological Reports, 65*, 643-647.

Examines age, gender, and personality correlates of self-actualization among 80 community men and women age 56-84. No main effect for gender is observed on Personal Orientation Inventory scores, but the elders (age 68-84) obtain lower scores than the younger respondents (age 56-67) on four subscales: existentiality, feeling reactivity, acceptance of aggression, and capacity for intimate contact.   The analysis shows, for men, inventory scores are positively associated with the traits of change and endurance and negatively correlated with abasement, order, and succorance. These findings suggest the components of self-actualization are differentially influenced by age for men and women and the traits accompanying self-actualization are gender-linked. [1.3]

<61> Ryff, C. D. (1982). Self-perceived personality change in adulthood and aging. *Journal of Personality and Social Psychology, 42*, 108-115.

Extends previous research on perceived changes in values among middle-age and older women and men. Data from 80 middle-age (40-55) and 80 older (60 and above) men and women reveal that middle-age and older women give instrumental values high priority when focusing on middle age than when focusing on old age. Men give lower preference to instrumental values (and higher priority to terminal values) for middle and old age. On developmental personality scales, older men have lower scores on achievement, dominance, and social recognition and higher scores on play. [1.3]

<62> Sinnott, J. D. (1982). Correlates of sex roles of older adults. *Journal of Gerontology, 37*, 587-594.

Discusses from a life span perspective how gender constructions seem based in a masculine framework, and the polarized gender roles are not so central to personality that they remained unchanged over the life span. Data from 369 community-dwelling elders investigate how older men and women classify themselves on sex role polarity or complexity. Femininity scores on the Bem Sex Role Inventory are higher for men and women in the older cohort, which is in accord with a shift toward femininity for older men. Elders who are polarized masculine report a number of factors in their life that set them apart from the androgynous--they are notably higher income, married men who have less life stress and visit physicians more frequently. [1.3, 6.2]

<63> Spiro, A. 3rd., Aldwin, C. M., Levenson, M. R., & Bosse, R.   (1990). Longitudinal findings from the Normative Aging Study: II. Do emotionality

and extroversion predict symptom change? *Journals of Gerontology: Psychological Sciences, 45*, P136-P144.

Investigates cross-sectionally and longitudinally how the personality traits of emotionality and extroversion are associated with symptoms among 1,034 men. The sample was initially screened for good health. Correlations reveal emotionality is positively related to the number of physical and psychological symptoms reported at baseline, whereas extroversion is negatively related. Once age is controlled, only emotionality is associated with symptom reporting. By comparison, longitudinal analyses reveal that emotionality is unrelated to physical symptoms and only weakly to psychological. Results suggest that although personality and symptom reporting are related cross-sectionally, personality does not predict changes in symptom reporting. [1.3, 2.4]

<64>   Turner, B. F. (1992). Gender differences in old age in ratings of aggression/assertiveness. *Current Psychology Research and Reviews, 11*, (2) 122-127.

Based on interview and paper-and-pencil test material on 60 elderly women and 25 elderly men, no gender differences are observed in personality ratings of aggression-assertiveness. Aggression is in women's accounts of current activities; in men, aggression is more often in their renditions of past-life activities. Findings are consistent with the possibility of age-related decline in aggression in men. [1.3]

<65>   West, R. L., Crook, T. H., & Barron, K. L. (1992). Everyday memory performance across the life span: Effects of age and noncognitive individual differences. *Psychology and Aging, 7*, 72-82.

Similar to others who examine the impact of individual-difference factors on memory, this study determines which individual-difference attributes--vocabulary, education, depression, gender, marital status, and employment status--mediate the effects of aging. Uses a sample of 2,495 adults age 18 to 90 and laboratory-analog tests of everyday memory. Age is consistently the most significant predictor, followed by verbal ability and gender. Men's disadvantage in memory may be test specific and a function of experience, since all five gender differences involve grocery lists and names. Findings affirm that individual differences can affect some memory test scores. [1.3]

<66>   Windle, M. (1986). Sex role orientation, cognitive flexibility, and life satisfaction among older adults. *Psychology of Women Quarterly, 10*, 263-273.

The relationships among gender orientation, cognitive flexibility, and life satisfaction in later life are examined among 34 older men and 67 older women using the Bem Sex Role Inventory. The categories masculine, feminine, and androgynous do not significantly differentiate older adults with respect to behavioral flexibility or life satisfaction. Further, in hierarchical regression analyses, neither masculinity, femininity, nor the interaction term (masculinity X femininity) are predictors of cognitive flexibility or life satisfaction. It is concluded that the median-split topological approach is of limited value for examining gender orientation in later adulthood. [1.3]

<67>   Windle, M., & Sinnott, J. D. (1985). Psychometric study of the Bem Sex
       Role Inventory with an older adult sample. *Journal of Gerontology, 40*,
       336-343.

Identifies the factorial structure and psychometric properties of the Bem Sex Role
Inventory among 364 senior center members. Confirmatory analysis reveal that the
two-factor model does not adequately represent the underlying factor structure for the
sample. The authors suggest that the structural component of masculinity and
femininity may differentiate with aging, yielding more than two dimensions. It is also
possible that patterns of personality reorganization in later life may vary with gender.
[1.3]

<68>   Zonderman, A. B., Siegler, I. C., Barefoot, J. C., Williams, R. B., Costa, P. T.
       Jr. (1993). Age and gender differences in the content scales of the Minne-
       sota Multiphasic Personality Inventory. *Experimental Aging Research, 19*,
       241-257.

Examines gender and age differences on the nine content scales of the Minnesota
Multiphasic Personality Inventory (MMPI). Data are from the 481 adults age 30-86 in
Baltimore Longitudinal Study of Aging, a study 3,722 undergraduates conducted at the
University of North Carolina, and a study of 2,050 male employees age 40-56 of
Western Electric Company. The findings show few age-related differences in the nine
content dimensions. Consistent gender differences are noted in two samples on three
of the nine content scales. Concludes that each gender should be examined separately
in future personality studies. [1.3]

LIFE COURSE EFFECTS ON SOCIAL ROLES

<69>   Adelmann, P. K. (1994). Multiple roles and psychological well-being in a
       national sample of older adults. *Journal of Gerontology: Social Sciences,
       49*, S277-S285.

Predicts multiple role involvement in late life is linked to greater psychological well-
being, based on activity theory and a role enhancement hypothesis. Using data on the
1,644 men and women age 60 and over from 1986 Americans' Changing Lives Survey,
finds that men hold fewer roles than women (employee, spouse, parent, volunteer,
homemakers, grandparent, caregiver, and student). Multiple roles are associated with
higher life satisfaction and self-efficacy, and the interaction terms with gender reveal the
effects of multiple roles are greater for men. The findings suggest men's role
involvement brings fewer burdens, and this is particularly true for older black men whose
late life roles may acquire greater importance after exclusion from regular employment.
[1.4, 2.3]

<70>   Allen, S. M., Mor, V., Raveis, V., & Houts, P. (1993). Measurement of need
       for assistance with daily activities: Quantifying the influence of gender
       roles. *Journals of Gerontology: Social Sciences, 48*, S204-S211.

Examines affect of gender expectations to receipt of assistance with personal care
activities, housekeeping, shopping, and transportation among a sample of 629 cancer

patients. Men (70 percent) name their wives as the person who helps most. Nearly 80 percent of the men (and 30 percent of the women) receive help with household tasks, and 80 percent of these men attribute help received with meal preparation, house-keeping and shopping to gender traditions and the division of labor within their established relationships. Adjusted estimates for underreporting of physical inability and overreporting of help reveals men's level of need for assistance is reduced from 80 to 37 percent. [1.4, 2.2, 7.5]

<71> Anderson, T. B. (1992). Conjugal support among working-wife and retired-wife couples. In M. Szinovacz, D. J. Ekerdt, & B. H. Vinick (Eds.), *Families and retirement* (pp. 175-188). Newbury Park, CA: Sage Publications.

Recognizes that most couples approaching retirement are dual-wage couples, and exit from the labor force may increase their interdependence. Examines the exchange of support between spouses. Finds no difference in emotional support and confiding among the older married couples -- husbands and wives in dual-employed, husband-only-retired, and dual-retired couples are similar in the extent to which they received support from and confided in their partner. Concludes that conjugal support is not a developmental task. [1.4, 7.5, 8.4]

<72> Elder, G. H., Shanahan, M. J., & Clipp, E. C. (1994). When war comes to men's lives: Life-course patterns in family, work, and health. *Psychology and Aging, 9,* 5-16.

Discusses how World War II expanded the period of service eligibility from age 18 to the late 30s. Hypothesizes that each year of delay adds greater risk of social disruption and its related costs, which ultimately result in adverse changes in adult health. Using data from the longitudinal Stanford Terman studies, finds late-mobilized men are at greatest risk of negative trajectories on physical health. Work-life disadvantages (e.g., interrupted careers, re-training) account in part for this health effect. [1.4]

<73> George, L. K., & Gold, D. T. (1991). Life course perspectives on intergen-erational and generational connections. *Marriage and Family Review, 16* (1-2), 67-88.

Evaluates the contributions and limitations of life course perspectives as conceptual tools for understanding generational and intergenerational connections in the family. Analyzes the impact of social change on family life course patterns during the past century, and determines that demographic and other changes generate new family forms and transform the parameters of family relationships. Discussion focuses on the verticalization of the family, age-condensed and age-gapped family structures, truncated family structures, reconstituted families, decreased involvement of men, the predictability of family transitions, and marital quality. [1.4, 6.2]

<74> Henretta, J. C., O'Rand, A. M., & Chan, C. G. (1993). Gender differences in employment after spouse's retirement. *Research on Aging, 15,* 148-169.

Theorizes retirement of one spouse in a two worker couple implies a reorganization of family roles as the couple begins the transition into retirement. Central to this two-worker family transition is its prolonged nature, beginning with the first spouse's retirement. Examines differences in the process using the 1982 Social Security New Beneficiary Study on men age 62-72. Hypothesizes that women would retire more rapidly following their husband's retirement because their labor force role is secondary to family roles. Finds no overall gender difference in the timing of men's and women's job exit or return rate, especially in couples with less segregated family roles. Concludes that trends toward earlier retirement for both men and women make the family retirement transition something of growing importance. [1.4, 10.2]

<75> Keith, P. M., Dobson, C. D., Goudy, W. J., & Powers, E. A. (1981). Older men: Occupation, employment status, household involvement, and well-being. *Journal of Family Issues, 2,* 336-349.

Evaluates the influence of occupation and employment status on the involvement of older men in the home. Data are from 1,193 married men age 60 or older who are employed, retired, or partially retired. Masculine and feminine household tasks are differentially effected by work status. Employed men are least involved in either type of task. Blue collar and salaried professionals are most involved among the five occupational groups, which challenges the curvilinear expectation that men in high- and low-status occupations would be least involved. Concludes that involvement in feminine tasks has little impact on men's sense of well-being, but participation in masculine activities is somewhat more salient to self and life evaluations. [1.4, 8.4]

<76> Miller, B. (1990). Gender differences in spouse caregiver strain: Socialization and role expectations. *Journal of Marriage and the Family, 52,* 311-321.

Examines two gender difference hypotheses--gender socialization vulnerability and social role exposure--to explain caregiver strains among the 554 spouse caregivers within the 1982 National Long Term Care Survey. Although men report lower levels of strain on two of three measures (time and health strains), gender effects occur only in health strain. Men report less. But the effect of gender is relatively small, suggesting gender difference models commonly used to explain findings for younger samples are not as useful in explaining later life findings. [1.4]

<77> Sinnott, J. D. (1984). Older men, older women: Are their perceived sex roles similar? *Sex Roles, 10,* 847-856.

Examines 364 older men's and women's views of their gender roles and their perceptions of social expectations about age-appropriate gender roles. They describe themselves and how other people expect them to be on the Bem Sex Role Inventory. Finds men and women report more similarly than difference for both masculine and feminine traits and concludes that the older adult cohort is generally androgynous. Conflicts between actual and expected attributes are more frequent on masculine items, particular for men. Men do not perceive as strong normative expectations as women. Elders who are most conflicted on masculine items report more recent life-event stress than their least-conflicted counterparts. [1.4, 2.3]

<78>   Spitze, G., & Logan, J. R. (1990). More evidence of women (and men) in the middle. *Research on Aging, 12,* 182-198.

Building on prior work, the authors reexamine the notion that it is middle-aged women who are often caught between multiple, stressful caregiving situations. Using a probability sample and presenting analyses for men's and women's involvement in major roles (spouse, paid work, adult child of aging parent, and parent), men are almost as likely as women to experience each role. When active involvement rather than simple occupancy of these roles is examined, much smaller percentages of men and women are combining work, parenting and parental caregiving. [1.4, 9.1]

<79>   Szinovacz, M., & Harpster, P. (1994). Couples' employment/retirement status and the division of household tasks. *Journals of Gerontology: Social Sciences, 49,* S125-S136.

Examines if the older couple's division of household labor and men's and women's housework contributions to traditionally male and female chores differ by their retirement status. From a subsample of the National Survey of Families and Households (N = 672), finds housework varies by gender and domain. Husbands' hours spent in female chores is a function of wives' employment status and his gender role traditionalism -- they perform more female housework if wives are employed, rather than retired or housewives. Nonparticipation is more common among husbands with traditional gender ideologies. The patterns demonstrate a need to understand both spouses' employment status and gender ideology. [1.4, 10.2]

ADULT DEVELOPMENT THEORY

<80>   Bennett, K. C., & Thompson, N. L. (1990). Accelerated aging and male homosexuality: Australian evidence in a continuing debate. *Journal of Homosexuality, 20* (3-4), 65-75.

Investigates the issue of accelerated aging among gay men. Questionnaire data from 478 homosexual men in Australia are used to compare how the onset of middle and old age is perceived personally and in terms of other men in the homosexual community. The duality of gay men's lifestyle as they interact in the homosexual community and the larger heterosexual society positively affects perceptions. Concludes that the contradictions about gay men and their accelerated aging are stereotypical thinking. [1.5]

<81>   Calasanti, T. M., & Zajicek, A. M. (1993). Socialist-feminist approach to aging: Embracing diversity. *Journal of Aging Studies, 7,* 117-131.

Presents a socialist-feminist approach to aging, with its focus on the historically and socially constructed nature of gender, class, and racial/ethnic relations. This approach embraces the diversity of experiences among the elderly. Conditions based on ageism and sexism cannot be ameliorated without knowledge of the relations of age and gender, especially the inequalities which often advantage men and disadvantage women. As argued, an inclusive research model embracing men and women needs to be used, not separate models for the two genders or a model that uses the experiences of men as the standard for women. [1.5]

<82>   Chodorow, N. J. (1986). Divorce, oedipal asymmetries, and the marital age gap. Special Issue: Toward a new psychology of men: Psychoanalytic and social perspectives. *Psychoanalytic Review, 73*, 606-610.

Proposes that oedipal asymmetries in male-female relationships result from growing up in families where mothers perform primary parenting functions and fathers are relatively absent. Theorizes that conflicting and ambivalent needs produce regularized tensions within men's heterosexual relationships. These tensions help account for rising divorce rates, and result in older men and older women reentering the marriage market. Age-hypergamous marriage provides men heterosexual intimacy and nurturance without threatening selfhood or generating too much dependence. Although an age-unequal male-female relationship seems to benefit both members, concludes that such a solution is socially and psychologically problematic. [1.5]

<83>   Feifel, H., & Strack, S. (1989). Coping with conflict situations: Middle-aged and elderly men. *Psychology and Aging, 4*, 26-33.

Reviews how old age involves far-reaching changes (e.g., body-image alterations, finances, developing a sense of the meaning of one's life); clinicians suggest that changes affect on how elders cope with stress. Investigates the coping responses of middle-aged (N = 76) and elderly men (N = 106) to five conflict situations--decision making, defeat in a competitive circumstance, frustration, authority conflict, and peer disagreement. Elderly men use avoidance less often than middle-aged men in handling decision making and authority-conflict situations; they use problem solving more than avoidance or resignation in all five conflict situations. Findings do not support clinicians who view men's aging in terms of withdrawal from gender norms, nor do they support developmentalist interpretations of coping. [1.5, 2.3, 6.2]

<84>   Florsheim, P., & Gutmann, D. L. (1992). Mourning the loss of "self as father": A longitudinal study of fatherhood among the Druze. *Psychiatry, 55*, 160-176.

Discusses how the psychodynamic effect of the adult child's independence of the aging father involves a loss for the older man of the "self as father." To the period of the adult child's separation, the father's adult life was largely devoted to providing. As children reach adulthood and no longer need parenting, among Druze men, this loss is felt most keenly. [1.5, 8.1]

<85>   Goldscheider, F. K. (1990). The aging of the gender revolution: What do we know and what do we need to know? *Research on Aging, 12*, 531-545.

Research on the elderly family has portrayed a warm network of kin ties, strong marital and family relationships. But this general image characterizes only the current population of elderly and near elderly, who have benefited from modernity. This group of elders are members of a deviant cohort who married young, had more children, and experienced greater marital continuity than any previous cohort. Cohorts soon entering old age in the 21st century will be different. Increasingly, the population we regard as "elderly" will reflect the labor force participation of women, the tremendous rise in divorce and childbearing outside marriage, the overall decline in marriage and remarriage, and the prevalence of old unmarried men. There will be cohorts of elders who have histories of family ties that are broken, weakened, and confused. Unlike previous generations, as employment-based resources become less central in old age and as family relationships grow in importance, it is males who are at risk. Even those who are remarried, many will have no relationship with their biological children. A number of important research directions are identified. [1.5, 6.2]

<86> Gutmann, D. L. (1987). *Reclaimed powers: Toward a new psychology of men and women in later life.* New York: Basic Books.

Proposes a new psychology of aging based on the development of new capacities in later life. Theorizes that older men and women come to possess psychological capacities previously unavailable to them. According to the theory, both men's and women's basic psychological potential is suppressed during the years they are fulfilling their distinct parental roles--providing versus nurturing. Once the child-rearing years are over, there is a passage to normal androgyny--men become more contemplative and expressive; women assume more assertive and competitive. This work includes research from the author's comparative studies of men in preliterate agricultural societies and ethnographic accounts covering a wide spectrum of cultures. [1.4, 1.5]

<87> Gutmann, D. L. (1986). Oedipus and the aging male: A comparative perspective. Special Issue: Toward a new psychology of men: Psychoanalytic and social perspectives. *Psychoanalytic Review, 73,* 541-552.

Proposes that men's aging can be discussed from the point of view of psychoanalytic inquiry. Comparing the treatment of elderly apes and that of the older men in primitive levels of human social organization (e.g., hunter-gatherers, preliterate folk-traditional societies), argues that as society moves away from participatory gerontocracy. The role of elder men as community superego and culture tenders erodes. Concludes that when patriarchal culture and the extended family are no longer tended by elder men, its replacement (the nuclear family) becomes fertile ground for forms of social pathology, particularly child abuse. [1.5]

<88> Kimmel, D. C. (1978). Adult development and aging: A gay perspective. *Journal of Social Issues, 34* (3), 113-130.

What happens to gay people when they grow older? To provide a model for understanding gay adult development and aging, Levinson's developmental scheme is applied to fourteen white, middle-class, well-educated gay men between the ages of 55 and 81 years. Although older gays may differ from younger gays, it is not clear whether these differences result from aging per se or from the different historical periods in which the individual had to deal with all that being a homosexual in our society entails. Older gays have special needs, such as support during bereavement, assistance if physically disabled, and a reduction in stigmatization. [1.5]

<89> Lowenthal, M. F., & Weiss, L. (1976). Intimacy and crises in adulthood. *Counseling Psychologist, 6,* 10-15.

Reports how the significance of interpersonal intimacy as a development task in adulthood--Erikson (1963)--has received little systematic study. Attributes the absence to the high degree of complexity and relativity of the concept of intimacy as well as the American male's traditional flight from intimacy. Hypothesizes that, in the absence of overwhelming external challenge, most individuals find the motivation to live autonomous and satisfying lives only through one or more mutually intimate dyadic relationships. Presents preliminary data in support of the hypothesis, and shows life stage and gender differences. Raises in discussion the implications of intimacy as a resource for middle-aged women in the post-maternal stage of life and middle-aged men who are overwhelmed by life stresses. [1.5]

<90> McAdams, D. P., de St. Aubin, E., & Logan R. L. (1993). Generativity among young, midlife, and older adults. *Psychology and Aging*, *8*, 221-230.

Conceptualizes generativity as a arrangement of psychosocial features organized around the goal of providing for the next generation. Uses a stratified random sample of young, midlife, and older (age 67-72) adults and examines age-cohort differences in four generativity features--generative concern, commitments, actions, and narration. Finds no significant differences for gender, just age-cohort. Nor is there any significant age by gender interaction. The age-cohort data demonstrate mid-life men and women score higher levels of generativity than young and older adults, and significantly higher than either age cohort at retest on generative concern and acts. These findings are interpreted as consistent with Erikson's model of development. [1.5]

<91> Pratt, M. W., Diessner, R., Hunsberger, B., Pancer, S. M., & Savoy, K. (1991). Four pathways in the analysis of adult development and aging: Comparing analyses of reasoning about personal-life dilemmas. *Psychology and Aging*, *6*, 666-675.

Compares the patterns of age differences in personal and social problem solving in a mid- to later-life sample using four systems--Kohlberg's moral judgment stages, Kegan's ego-development stages, Gilligan's moral orientation system, and Suedfeld and Tetlock's integrative complexity scoring. Data are the personal-life dilemmas discussed by 29 men and 35 women (ages 35-85). Finds no significant differences across mid- to later adulthood in reasoning about personal dilemmas, once educational background is controlled. This suggests no added development nor "regression" in later-life social and moral reasoning. No gender differences in Kohlberg's average justice levels, Kegan's stages, but differences are present on the Gilligan orientation index. Men more likely use justice-type reasoning rather than care-oriented reasoning. These differences could be accounted for by the types of dilemmas produced by the two sexes, with men less likely to recount personal relationship problems. [1.3, 1.5]

<92> Shimonaka, Y., Nakazato, K., & Marushima, R. (1994). Androgyny and psychological well-being among older and younger Japanese adults. *Aging*, *6*, 43-48.

Examines Gutmann's role reversal theory and Sinnott's role blurring (androgyny) theory using a sample of 384 Japanese community elders, compared to 289 students. The Bem Sex Role Inventory is used to measure gender orientation. Finds masculinity is higher among men than women, and the older showed higher femininity than the young.

However, no significant cohort by gender interaction is observed in either masculine or feminine scores. Androgynous men and women possess higher self-esteem. The results support Sinnott but not Gutmann. [1.5]

<93> Sinnott, J. D. (1977). Sex-role inconstancy, biology, and successful aging: A dialectical model. *The Gerontologist, 17,* 459-463.

Examines gender-role inconstancy from a life-span point of view. Theorizes that new environmental realities and an increasing life-span may make traditional gender roles less functional in old age. Evidence is presented for more successful aging in persons manifesting convergent gender-role behavior. A dialectical model is utilized to show how synthesis of conflicting role demands in the biological, cultural, and psychological spheres may be adaptive. [1.5]

<94> Thomas, L. E. (1991). Dialogues with three religious renunciates and reflections on wisdom and maturity. *International Journal of Aging and Human Development, 32,* 211-227.

In-depth interviews and participation observation with elderly Hindu religious renunciates living in India indicate that the elders are highly mature by Western developmental models, but known Western correlates of life satisfaction are not found. Implications for Western aging are discussed, particularly the importance of contemplation and acceptance of death. [1.5, 6.2]

<95> Thompson, E. H. (1994). Older men as invisible men in contemporary society. In E. Thompson (Ed.), *Older men's lives* (pp. 1-21). Thousand Oaks, CA: Sage Publications.

Discusses older men's invisibility in the family studies and gerontology literatures, and critiques the homogenizing of older men into the genderless categories of "elders" or "aged males." Argues what distinguishes older men is their cohort-specific, gendered social lives. What distinguishes them from older women, research shows, is their relatively advantaged social lives in terms of what incomes, independent living arrangements, and marital status offer. What distinguishes them from middle-age and younger men is theoretically equivocal and unexplored. [1.4, 1.5]

<96> White, C. B. (1988). Age, education, and sex effects on adult moral reasoning. *International Journal of Aging and Human Development, 27,* 271-281.

Utilizing Kohlberg's cognitive-developmental stage theory, examines the effects of age and education in adult moral reasoning. Interviews are with 195 adults age 19 to 92, and ranging in years of education from 3 to 25. No overall effect for age or sex is present, but there is an effect for education. Gender is not a significant predictor of moral reasoning at least partially due to educational differences. Men in this sample have higher overall education levels, and it is not possible to totally isolate the separate contributions of gender and education. Older men, however, do not reveal a different cognitive/moral stage than younger adults. In separate regression analyses for men and for women, however, age is not a predictor. [1.3, 1.5]

2

Health and Well-Being

— ♦ —

AGING AND PHYSICAL HEALTH

<97> Alterman, T., Shekelle, R. B., Vernon, S. W., & Burau, K. D. (1994). Decision latitude, psychologic demand, job strain, and coronary heart disease in the Western Electric Study. *American Journal of Epidemiology, 139*, 620-627.

Investigates the hypothesis that low decision latitude and high psychological demand are associated with increased risk coronary heart disease death. Data are from a 25-year follow-up study of 1,683 men age 38-56 in the Western Electric Study (1957-1983). After adjustment for coronary risk factors, the relative risk for 25-year coronary death was 0.76 for a decision latitude, 0.78 for the psychological demand, and 1.40 for job strain (defined by low decision latitude and high psychological demand). Analysis indicate that the effect of decision latitude is more pronounced for white-collar than for blue-collar workers. However, there is only limited evidence for associations between job characteristics and coronary heart disease mortality. [2.1, 2.3]

<98> Arbuckle, T. Y., Gold, D. P., Andres, D., Schwartzman, A., & Chaikelson, J. S. (1992). The role of psychosocial context, age, and intelligence in memory performance of older men. *Psychology and Aging, 7*, 25-36.

Hypothesizes that psychosocial contexts contribute to developmental changes in memory. The availability of data on 326 male World War II veterans' intelligence scores as young adults make it possible to separate from their performance on 4 memory tasks the effects of contextual variables and age on maintenance of general intelligence. Being healthier, more introverted, educated, intellectually active, satisfied with social support, and younger predict less intellectual decline and, indirectly, better memory performance. Concludes that personality, age, and the extent of social support contribute to performance on 1 or more memory tasks. [1.5, 2.1]

<99> Ashworth, J. B., Reuben, D. B., & Benton, L. A. (1994). Functional profiles of healthy older persons. *Age and Ageing, 23*, 34-39.

Monitors younger (25 men and 21 women) and older adults (21 men and 23 women) participating in a study on normative aging of the cardiovascular system. Examines whether the percentage of time spent at different functional levels varies as a function of age. For a single 24-hour weekday, the men and women are fitted with an ambulatory blood pressure monitor and a digital recorder monitoring heart rate, skin temperature, and core temperature, and they keep a activity diary. Older persons spend larger percentages of their day performing basic activities of daily living--10.9 percent versus 6.6 percent--and instrumental activities of daily living--9.8 percent versus 7.5 percent. The differences reflect primarily the difference between older and younger women. Older men more closely resemble young men. Concludes that gender expectations rather than age may be a more prominent factor in determining functional profiles in healthy older persons. [2.1, 2.2]

<100> Barrett-Conner, E., & Wingard, D. L. (1991). Heart disease risk factors as determinants of dependency and death in an older cohort: The Rancho Bernardo study. *Journal of Aging and Health, 3,* 247-261.

Determines rates of dependency and death in a cohort of 621 older upper-class, white adults who are initially interviewed between 1972 and 1974. Between 1984 and 1986, participants or their next-of-kin are reinterviewed. Finds dependency prior to death for 71 percent of the men who died during the follow-up period and for 86 percent of the women who died. Dependency rates increase with age for men, not for women, and rates for men and women are highest in the year before death. Age, presence of chronic disease, and (in women) lack of siblings predict death and dependency. [2.1, 7.5]

<101> Bowling, A. (1987). Mortality after bereavement: A review of the literature on survival periods and factors affecting survival. *Social Science and Medicine, 24,* 117-124.

Reviews research on mortality after bereavement, noting that mortality rates for widowed people in every age group are higher than for married people. The research also suggests that the excess risk is greater for men. Little is known, however, about the causes of their apparently higher mortality rates. [2.1, 2.3]

<102> Bryant, S., & Rakowski, W. (1992). Predictors of mortality among elderly African Americans. *Research on Aging, 14,* 50-67.

Finds that for the 330 female and 185 male elderly African-Americans in the 1984-1988 Longitudinal Survey of Aging age 70 and older, lower mortality is associated with three indices of informal social networks--contacts with family members, contacts with friends, and social involvement outside the home. Church attendance is significant to lower mortality in a logistic regression equation controlling for self-rated health, physical health and sociodemographic variables. Men appear to be at high risk when their social network is limited. [2.1, 5.1]

<103> Christensen, K. J., Moye, J., Armson, R. R., & Kern, T. M. (1992). Health screening and random recruitment for cognitive aging research. *Psychology and Aging, 7,* 204-208.

Discusses how the health status of elders generally fails to consider cognitive status during sample recruitment. Analysis of 197 studies of cognitive aging finds infrequent use of screening health assessments. On the basis of self-reported medical problems, one third of the subjects initially contacted would be excluded. They are more likely to be older and men. Subjects who pass screening and choose to participate in neuropsychological research project are younger, better educated, and also more often men than nonparticipants. Concludes that attention to health status and gender bias in sampling is needed. [2.1, 12.1]

<104> Clark, D. O., & Maddox, G. L. (1992). Racial and social correlates of age-related changes in functioning. *Journals of Gerontology: Social Sciences, 47*, S222-S232.

Examines social and racial differences in age-related functioning across a decade for a panel of 566 black and 5,196 non-blacks in the Longitudinal Retirement History Survey. "Functioning" is measured as physical functioning, self-care capacity, and self-rated well-being. Trajectories largely vary in the expected manner, and they are not linear. Unexpectedly, non-black men on average display higher levels of functional impairment than women when poverty status is held constant. Age changes do not differ across racial groups, as would be predicted by the multiple-jeopardy hypothesis. [2.1]

<105> Clipp, E. C., Pavalko, E. K., & Elder, G. H. (1991-92). Trajectories of health: In concept and empirical pattern. *Behavior, Health, and Aging, 2*, 159-179.

Based on original surveys by Terman (1925), the health histories of 857 men are reexamined to identify broad patterns of stability and change in health between 1940 and 1986. Qualitative data analysis describe trajectories characteristic of most individuals, and quantitative analysis differentiate these patterns using individual and medical characteristics. This approach focuses on the sequence of health transitions, and provides methodological and substantive insights regarding physical and emotional processes. [2.1]

<106> Cohen, C. I., Teresi, J. A., & Holmes, D. (1988). The physical well-being of old homeless men. *Journals of Gerontology: Social Sciences, 43*, S121-S128.

Compares 195 nonstreet dwelling men age 50 and older residing in "flophouses," 86 homeless street dwellers, and aged-matched community men for the etiology, prevalence, and treatment of physical disorders among aging homeless men.. Shows the men on skid row have significantly worse physical health, particularly in the disease categories comprising the "skid row syndrome"--lung disease, hypertension, gastrointestinal disease, and physical trauma. Less than one in every five of homeless men perceive their health as poor, yet stress, unfulfilled needs, alcohol abuse, seeking help from community agencies, and depressed affect are all associated with poor health. The poor health appears to antedate arrival on the Bowery. [2.1, 10.1]

<107> Costa, P. T. Jr., & McCrae, R. R. (1980). Somatic complaints in males as a function of age and neuroticism: A longitudinal analysis. *Journal of Behavioral Medicine, 3*, 245-257.

Investigates the influence of age and neuroticism on reports of physical complaints in various bodily systems using 6- and 12-year longitudinal analyses of the physical health from a group of 1,038 men in the Baltimore Longitudinal Study of Aging. Finds problems in sensory, cardiovascular, and genitourinary symptoms increase with age, while health habits improve. Results suggest that age does not produce a generalized increase in physical complaints; instead, specific age-related symptoms show increases. [1.3, 2.1]

<108> Curb, J. D., Reed, D. M., Miller, F. D., & Yano, K. (1990). **Health status and life style in elderly Japanese men with a long life expectancy.** *Journals of Gerontology: Social Sciences, 45,* S206-S211.

Investigates the health status and life style characteristics of the population Japanese and Chinese men living in Hawaii, who are among the longest lived of any group of males in the U.S. Data are on 1,379 community-dwelling men age 60-81, and the findings reveal the prevalence of major limitations of mobility is relatively low. Less than one percent of these men rate their health status as poor, and the number who live alone is also low. Concludes with a discussion of life style affects on longevity. [2.1,]

<109> Ekerdt, D. J., Bosse, R., & LoCastro, J. S. (1983). **Claims that retirement improves health.** *Journal of Gerontology, 38,* 231-236.

Uses prospective data to compare men (N = 114) who claim that retirement had a good effect on their health with men (N = 149) who claim that retirement had no effect on their health. Finds the retrospective claims of good effects are not corroborated by a corresponding longitudinal (pre- to postretirement) improvement in self-reported health. Claims of good effects are more likely among men whose retirement entails the reduction of prior job strain and role demands. This finding supports the interpretation that good health claims represent the enhancement of functional health status. [2.1, 10.2]

<110> Elder, G. H. (1991). **Making the best of life: Perspectives on lives, times, and aging.** *Generations, 15* (1), 12-17.

Summarizes several longitudinal studies which find that the people who make the best out of life are frequently those who have managed to surmount earlier disadvantages. Three longitudinal studies--the Berkeley Growth Study, the Berkeley Guidance Study (birth years, 1928-1929), and the Oakland Growth Study (birth years 1920-1921)--followed adults from middle and working class backgrounds to later life in the 1980s. The grew up in the Depression, experienced the mobilization of World War II, and followed careers to later life in a more affluent postwar era. For a large number of men impaired by family conditions in the 1930s, military mobilization during the 1940s pulled them into a more promising trajectory and enabled many to make the best of their lives, equipping them for aging well after retirement. [1.4, 2.1, 4.4]

<111> Falk, A., Hanson, B. S., Isacsson, S. O., & Ostergren, P. O. (1992). **Job strain and mortality in elderly men: Social network, support, and influence as buffers.** *American Journal of Public Health, 82,* 1136-1139.

Investigates whether exposure to job strain during the active working period affects mortality in elderly men after retirement, and whether social network and support outside the place of work can buffer the negative health effects of job strain. Data are on 477 men born in Malmo, Sweden in 1914. Exposure to job strain increases the mortality risk after retirement. The combination of exposure to job strain and weak social support in retirement is associated with a further increase in relative mortality risk. [2.1, 2.3, 7.5, 10.2]

<112> Ferraro, K. F. (1987). **Double jeopardy to health for older black adults.** *Journal of Gerontology, 42,* 528-533.

Prior health research on the double disadvantage of being black and old is based on subjectively defined health. Examines the double jeopardy thesis with subjective and objective health measures from a national sample of 3,183 older adults. After controlling for objective health conditions, finds older blacks tend to have poorer health, are more limited in daily functioning by their health problems, and evaluate their own health more negatively . Black men manifest more health optimism than black women, maybe because surviving older black men are an elite who have lived beyond the age of cohort peers. The double jeopardy hypothesis is not supported, because the white-black gap in health does not widen with age. [2.1, 2.4]

<113> Forster, L. E., & Stoller, E. P. (1992). **The impact of social support on mortality: A seven-year follow-up of older men and women.** *Journal of Applied Gerontology, 11,* 173-186.

Examines the impact of social support on 7-year survival rates of 363 elderly community residents whose average age 73 at the time of the first interview. One-third had died at 7-year follow-up. There is a positive relationship between social integration as a measure of social support and survival. Regardless of health status, being connected to the social world via roles and responsibilities provides elders, especially the women, with a survival advantage. [2.1, 7.5, 7.1]

<114> Fries, J. F., Williams, C. A., & Morfeld, D. (1992). **Improvement in intergenerational health.** *American Journal of Public Health, 81,* 109-112.

Compares the health status among 2,206 elders who had attended the University of Pennsylvania during 1939-1940, their patients, and their children. Elders compared their own health status at the average age of 70 (in 1988) with that of their same-sex patent at the same age (approximately in 1963) and with that of their same-sex child who is approximately 45. More than half of the older men and two-thirds of the women define their health as better than that of their parents at the same age, because of healthier life styles and the decreased prevalence of chronic conditions. Finds virtually identical results in a community-based sample of another 317 elders. Both samples suggest the average age of infirmity is delayed and the amount of life spent infirmed is decreasing. [2.1]

<115> Gallagher, E. (1990). **Emotional, social, and physical health characteristics of older men in prison.** *International Journal of Aging and Human Development, 31,* 251-265.

Compares the social, emotional, and physical health characteristics of inmates in three medium-security Federal prisons in Canada. When compared with younger inmates, the older men have more contacts with friends and family more friends in prison, and experience less stress than the younger men. Further, their physical health does not appear to be any worse when compared to the young men. [2.1, 2.2, 11.1]

<116> Hanson, B. S., & Ostergren, P. O. (1987). **Different social network and social support characteristics, nervous problems and insomnia: Theoretical and methodological aspects of some results from the population study 'Men born in 1917', Malmo, Sweden.** *Social Science and Medicine, 25,* 849-859.

Examines the effects of social network, social support and social influence on men's health status in a representative sample of Swedish men age 68. Men living alone and men in the lowest social class have the most insufficient social networks and social support and greater morbidity. Using structural indices of network, prior findings are replicated. Men with nervous problems had weaker social anchorage, lower contact frequency and more inadequate social participation and emotional support. [2.1, 7.5]

<117> Haug, M. R., & Folmar, S. J. (1986). **Longevity, gender, and life quality.** *Journal of Health and Social Behavior, 27,* 332-345.

Reports the effects of men's shorter life expectancy on their quality of life. Longitudinal data are from the U.S. General Accounting Office study of 647 Cleveland, Ohio elders. Three cohorts of elderly -- those age 65 to 74, 75 to 84, and 85 and older in 1975 -- are interviewed, and survivors are reinterviewed in 1984. Not unexpectedly, the sample is two-thirds women. Men generally experience a better quality of life according to all the indicators used. Gender differences in living alone and in activities of daily living are most visible, and men are more advantaged. Assessment of changes reveal that aging rather than cohort membership accounts for variations. Both gender and age affect cognitive ability, self-rated health, and functional ability, even when other demographic factors are controlled. Discusses the findings in terms of theories of active life expectancy and the compression of morbidity. [2.1, 2.4, 2.5]

<118> Herzog, A. R., House, J. S., & Morgan, J. N. (1991). **Relation of work and retirement to health and well-being in older age.** *Psychology and Aging, 6,* 202-211.

Reviews what little is known about the impact of work activity on health and well-being among older Americans. Studies patterns of labor-force participation and an array of physical and psychological well-being indicators. Finds that the sheer amount of work has little relationship to health and well-being. As hypothesized, persons whose patterns of labor-force participation reflect their personal preference report higher levels of physical and psychological well-being than those whose participation (or nonparticipation) is constrained by other factors. Results do not differ by gender. [2.1, 2.3, 10.2]

<119> Johnson, R. J., & Wolinsky, F. D. (1994). **Gender, race, and health: The structure of health status among older adults.** *The Gerontologist, 34,* 24-35.

Examines a model of the structure of health status--one which includes disease, disability, functional limitation, and perceived health--for possible race and/or gender biases. The model proposes that the major impact of disease on perceived health is mediated by disability and functional limitation. Data confirm the structure of the model, and it varies significantly by gender. Discusses how among men, household activities in daily living lack predictive validity, which in turn strongly suggests that the traditional ADL scales might also lack predictive validity for men because the scales emphasize household tasks (such as cleaning and meal preparation). Concludes that measures of lower body disability contain items that are valid with regard to race and gender, but other ADL measures exhibit noncomparable race and gender differences. [2.1, 2.2]

<120> Kaufman, A. S., Kaufman-Packer, J. L., McLean, J. E., & Reynolds, C. R. (1991). Is the pattern of intellectual growth and decline across the adult life span different for men and women?. *Journal of Clinical Psychology,* 47, 801-812.

Comparisons on the WAIS-R for 1,480 adults ages 20-74 years are made to determine whether men and women differ in their age-related patterns of change on tests of fluid and crystallized abilities. Examining age by gender interactions, finds the interactions are basically nonsignificant and trivial. Both men and women maintain their crystallized abilities through old age and experience early, rapid declines in fluid ability. Discusses the results in terms of prior work on aging, gender, and cognitive abilities. [1.1, 1.3]

<121> Keil, J. E., Sutherland, S. E., Knapp, R. G., & Tyroler, H. A. (1992). Does equal socioeconomic status in black and white men mean equal risk of mortality? *American Journal of Public Health,* 82, 1133-1136.

Mortality studies focus on ethnicity and race and trigger concerns that mortality is greater among blacks because of race. Hypothesizes that when socioeconomic status is adequately considered, black-white mortality inequalities would be insignificant. Using the Charleston Heart Study of black and white men who were 35 to 74 in 1960, education level and occupational status are set as baseline, rather than race. Compare mortality over the ensuing 28 years. In no instance are black-white differences in all-cause or coronary disease mortality rate significantly different when controlled for socioeconomic status. [2.1]

<122> Kozma, A., Stones, M. J., & Hanna, T. E. (1991). Age, activity, and physical performance: An evaluation of performance models. *Psychology and Aging,* 6, 43-49.

Evidence exists for the relationship among age, physical activity, and performance. Assesses the better explanation for this persistent relationship across five age cohorts involving more than 6,000 people who range in age from 20 to 69. No support is found for the postulate that physical activity and age interact to determine functional capacity. Rather, larger age differences in four of five performance domains for men than women are evidenced, which means men may age more rapidly than women. [2.1, 2.4]

<123> Larrabee, G. J., & Crook, T. H. (1993). Do men show more rapid age-associated decline in simulated everyday verbal memory than do women? *Psychology and Aging, 8,* 68-71.

Magnetic resonance imaging data suggests that men show more rapid age-associated atrophy of the left hemisphere than do women. Investigated whether a similar pattern occurs for functional decline, testing 417 male-female pairs, age 17-79, matched on age and education. Age and gender directly effect performance -- older subjects and men perform more poorly on the three tests. Also finds just one of 15 age-by-gender interactions significant. Concludes that although men undergo more rapid decline in rate of left hemisphere structural decline with normal aging, these differences do not translate into differential functional decline in verbal learning and memory. [1.3, 2.1]

<124> Lee, D. J., & Markides, K. S. (1990). Activity and mortality among aged persons over an eight year period. *Journals of Gerontology: Social Sciences, 45,* S39-S42.

Examines the influence of level of activity on mortality with data from an eight-year (1976-1984) longitudinal study of 508 older Mexican Americans and Anglos. When age, gender, education, marital status, ethnicity, and self-rated health are controlled in the analysis, level of activity is not a significant predictor of mortality. The lack of association appears due to age, not gender or the other sociodemographic characteristics. [2.1, 7.1]

<125> Maddox, G. L., & Clark, D. O. (1992). Trajectories of functional impairment in later life. *Journal of Health and Social Behavior, 33,* 114-125.

Documents the late adulthood age-related trajectories of functional impairment that emerge over a decade. Data are from the Longitudinal Retirement History Study. Finds nonlinear trajectories are common. An initial association between being a man and lower rates of impairment disappears and is reversed when education and income are introduced in the analysis. Analysis of the relationships among gender, socioeconomic status, and functional impairment across the decade strongly suggests that in health research, there is limited usefulness to broad characterizations of impairment among "the" elder or among "older men." Work must begin addressing the interaction of social and biological factors since gender and SES are broad, crude proxy variables. [2.1]

<126> Manton, K. G. (1988). A longitudinal study of functional change and mortality in the United States. *Journals of Gerontology: Social Sciences, 43,* S153-S161.

Directly examines the individual transitions into and out of functionally impaired states using longitudinal data from the 1982 and 1984 National Long Term Care Surveys. There are significant numbers of community residents who apparently manifest long-term improvement in functioning, and the risks of becoming disabled are roughly the same for men and women. These findings suggest that gender differences in the national prevalence of disabilities arise from the greater longevity of women at any given level of age and functional impairment. [2.1, 2.2]

<127> **Metter, E. J., Walega, D., Metter, E. L., Pearson, J., Brant, L. J., Hiscock, B. S., & Fozard, J. L. (1992). How comparable are healthy 60- and 80-year-old men?** *Journals of Gerontology: Medical Sciences, 47,* M73-M78.

Cross-sectional research assumes that healthy 60-year-old men are equivalent to healthy 80-year-old men, but the comparability of different age men is largely unknown. To examine this issue, 212 healthy men age 60 are identified and 61 followed to age 80 in the Baltimore Longitudinal Study of Aging. Compared to a group of healthy 80-year-olds, the followed group have more heart disease, cancer, stroke, arterial, digestive, and peripheral nervous system diseases, and just 27 of the 61 continue to be healthy. Systolic pressure and serum cholesterol at age 60 are predictive of who would be healthy at age 80. [2.1, 2.2]

<128> **Meyers, D. A., Goldberg, A. P., Bleecker, M. L., Coon, P. J., Drinkwater, D. T., & Bleecker, E. R. (1991). Relationship of obesity and physical fitness to cardiopulmonary and metabolic function in healthy older men.** *Journals of Gerontology: Medical Sciences, 46,* M57-M65.

Determines the relationship of obesity and physical fitness to cardiopulmonary and metabolic function (or the "rate of aging"). Concludes that while age affects the cardiopulmonary and metabolic function of obese older men, physical inactivity, obesity, and an abdominal body fat distribution contribute significantly to their reductions in physiological function. [2.1]

<129> **Mitsuhashi, T. (1988). Study of the health of the elderly from the standpoint of Shinto.** *Journal of Religion and Aging, 4,* 127-131.

Reviews aspects of the Shinto lifestyle that are conducive to physical, mental, and social well-being in old age. As argued, the fundamental problem of late life is to promote and preserve health, despite the nearness of death. The Japanese Shinto religion is based on ceremonial rites and festivals that are repeated annually to ensure the renewal of life, thereby emphasizing the cyclical relationship between life and death. Shinto recognizes that all natural objects and phenomena have the same spirits as men; coexisting with these natural elements seems to relieve the loneliness of the elderly. Japanese respect and coexist with their ancestors through the Shinto lifestyle. [2.1, 5.2]

<130> **Moore, D. E., & Hayward, M. D. (1990). Occupational careers and mortality of elderly men.** *Demography, 27,* 31-53.

Uses the event histories of 3,080 men from the National Longitudinal Survey of Mature Men to examine occupational differentials in mortality among men age 55 years and older in the United States during the period 1966-1983. The known socioeconomic differentials in mortality are examined by studying the differential effects of occupation over the career cycle. Hazard-models show that the mortality of current or last occupation differs substantially from that of longest occupation, controlling for education, income, health status, and sociodemographic factors. The rate of mortality is reduced by the complexity of the longest occupation while social skills and physical and environmental demands of the latest occupation lower mortality. [2.1, 10.2]

<131> Nathan, R. J., Laffey, P., Lord, G., & Weiss, B. (1983). **Normal psychology of the aging male: Normal elderly men: A longitudinal study.** *Journal of Geriatric Psychiatry, 16,* 163-188.

Summarizes findings of a longitudinal study on changes occurring in white, elderly men's psychological and physical status, degree of brain atrophy, and ability to live independently in the community. The men are in worse shape physically than a sample of women when examined by an internist, however when evaluated by the OARS examiner, the men appear to be healthier -- their mental health, cognitive abilities, and some concentration abilities show better performance. The critical part of the study, the brain scan, shows men are more affected than are women of a comparable age. Discussion addresses reasons for this apparent association of good psychological and social adjustment with greater brain atrophy among the men. [2.1, 2.2]

<132> Ouslander, J. G., & Abelson, S. (1990). **Perceptions of urinary incontinence among elderly outpatients.** *The Gerontologist, 30,* 369-376.

Examines the perceptions of urinary incontinence among 164 women and 35 men (mean age = 78) who had been referred to an outpatient continence clinic. The older men and women do not differ in the view that urinary incontinence is inconvenient, embarrassing, or distressing, and more than one-third say it significantly interferes with their daily lives. Amount rather than frequency of urinary loss is associated with negative perceptions. [2.1, 2.2]

<133> Poehlman, E. T., Melby, C. L., & Badylak, S. F. (1991). **Relation of age and physical exercise status on metabolic rate in younger and older healthy men.** *Journals of Gerontology: Biological Sciences, 46,* B54-B58.

Little is known regarding the effect of regular participation in physical exercise on metabolic rate in aging men. Examines the influence of age and habitual physical exercise level on resting metabolic rate and thermic effect of a meal test (TEM) in physically active and sedentary younger and older men. Finds TEM is highest in active younger and active older men. A sedentary life style in older men may be associated with lower resting metabolic rate and its dangers. [2.1, 2.5]

<134> Rakowski, W., & Mor, V. (1992). **The association of physical activity with mortality among older adults in the Longitudinal Study of Aging (1984-1988).** *Journals of Gerontology: Medical Sciences, 47,* M122-M129.

Examines self-reported physical activity or exercise and mortality among 5,901 adults (2,222 men) age 70 and older using the Longitudinal Study of Aging. For the whole sample, not getting enough exercise or not having a regular exercise routine is associated with a higher risk of mortality. For men, it is the judgments made about their activity levels (e.g., activity compared to age peers, or the feeling of not getting enough exercise) which are predictive, not the behaviors themselves. Physicians should attend to reports of activity level as one of the broader psychosocial domains. [2.1, 2.5, 12.2]

<135> Rediehs, M. H., Reis, J. S., & Creason, N. S. (1990). **Sleep in old age: Focus on gender differences.** *Sleep, 13,* 410-424.

Meta-analysis of 27 studies of gender differences on 31 indices of sleep continuity, architecture, and pathology reveals elderly men have greater objective sleep pathologies than elderly women and greater variability from the patterns of health youthful sleep. Subjectively, cultural imperatives to be strong and capable may inhibit men from recognizing or admitting sleep problems. Results underscore the importance of health providers having an understanding of gender and age in relation to sleep. [2.1, 12.2]

<136> **Rogers, R. G., Rogers, A., & Belanger, A. (1992). Disability-free life among the elderly in the United States: Sociodemographic correlates of functional health.** *Journal of Aging and Health, 4,* **19-42.**

Determines the sociodemographic factors associated with length and quality of life. Logit analysis of data on 3,202 elders in the Longitudinal Study of Aging finds increasing age predictive of functional disability and a poor prognosis for recovery, except among older black men. Disability level and its predictors substantially vary by race and sex groups, demanding separate analyses for each subpopulation. Discusses how gender role differences influence reporting of disability, and how rates reflect cultural factors rather than true disabilities. [2.1]

<137> **Rushing, B., Ritter, C., & Burton, R. P. (1992). Race differences in the effects of multiple roles on health: Longitudinal evidence from a national sample of older men.** *Journal of Health and Social Behavior, 33,* **126-139.**

Examines longitudinally the effects of social roles (employment, marriage, and being a supporter) on health limitations and mortality for 1,845 white and 607 black men. Data are from the older men cohort of the National Longitudinal Surveys of Labor Market Experience. The men were age 55-69 at the initial assessment. Finds social roles continue to be associated with fewer health limitations in later life. Employment has the most consistent health-protective effect, and the benefits of employment are more pronounced for older black men than for whites. Marriage affects health in conjunction with employment. These results illustrate the importance of ascribed statuses as structural determinants of the relationship between roles and health. [2.1, 2.3]

<138> **Schaie, K. W. (1989). The hazards of cognitive aging.** *The Gerontologist, 29,* **484-493.**

Draws on the Seattle Longitudinal Study's five panels, applies an event history analysis to data involving changes (or declines) in states of individuals' cognitive abilities. The research is interested in when cognitive abilities change--do they change uniformly through adulthood or are there different life-course patterns? Findings reveal no uniform pattern of age-related changes across all intellectual abilities. Although fluid abilities tend to decline earlier than crystallized abilities, there are substantial gender differences as well. Men decline less rapidly on active or fluid abilities than women, but men may decline earlier on passive or crystallized abilities. [2.1]

<139> **Schoefeld, D. E., Malmrose, L. C., Blazer, D. G., Gold, D. T., & Seeman, T. E. (1994). Self-rated health and mortality in the high-functioning elderly. A closer look at healthy individuals: MacArthur Field Study of successful aging.** *Journals of Gerontology: Medical Sciences, 49,* **M109-M115.**

Theorizes that subjective health may be an especially important component among eldgers, since they are prone to multiple health problems which include not only physical components but psychological and social ones as well. Data from the MacArthur Field Study (457 men and 580 women age 70-79 at baseline) are use to examine the hypothesis. Findings affirm the hypothesis -- subjective health is the most predictive variable of mortality in controlled analyses, with gender (men's early deaths) consistently present. Health care professionals should be sensitive to the significance of poor self-rated health in apparently healthy patients. [2.1, 2.4]

<140> Seeman, T. E., Charpentier, P. A., Berkman, L. F., Tinetti, M. E., Guralnik, J. M., Albert, M., Blazer, D. G., & Rowe, J. W. (1994). Predicting changes in physical performance in a high-functioning elderly cohort: MacArthur Studies of successful aging. *Journals of Gerontology: Medical Sciences*, *49*, M97-M108.

Challenges the perceived inevitability of age-related decreases in functional ability, and examines three-year changes in physical performance of 1,192 men and women age 70-79 using performance-based measures. Finds a wide range of performance abilities in a cohort initially selected for relatively high levels of functioning. At baseline, men, whites, those with higher education and income, and those with fewer chronic conditions reveal better performance ability. Declines are predicted by older age, lower income, weight and blood pressure, and incidence of health problems, yet declines are neither inevitable nor uniformly negative. Improvements are not uncommon--the majority maintained or improved their relatively high levels of functioning. [2.1]

<141> Stanford, E. P., Happersett, C. J., Morton, D. J., Molgaard, C. A., & Peddecord, K. M. (1991). Early retirement and functional impairment from a multi-ethnic perspective. *Research on Aging*, 13, 5-38.

Compares self-reported health measures and objective functional impairment ratings for the early retired and the nonretired among three ethnic groups -- whites, blacks, and Mexican-Americans. Functional impairment is higher among men who retire early and is predictive of early retirement for the men in the three ethnic groups. Mexican-American men have the greatest variety of factors contributing to early retirement status. [2.1, 10.2]

<142> Tenover, J. S., & Bremner, W. J. (1991). Circadian rhythm of serum immunoreactive inhibin in young and elderly men. *Journals of Gerontology: Medical Sciences*, 46, M181-M184.

Examines whether serum immunoreactive inhibin levels demonstrate a circadian variation in young men and if normal aging has an effect on the 24-hour serum inhibin pattern. Hourly blood samples are obtained for 24 hours from 7 young men (age 25-35) and 7 elderly men (age 65-72). Similar to testosterone, serum inhibin levels demonstrated a circadian pattern. Elderly men presented a circadian rhythm in serum inhibin, with an average amplitude that is not significantly different from that found in young men. However, the average 24-hour inhibin level in the elderly men is significantly lower than is found in young men. These patterns affirm immunoreactive inhibin displays a rhythm in the serum of adult men, and the inhibin biorhythm is maintained in elderly men. [2.1]

<143> Thorslund, M., & Lundberg, O. (1994). **Health and inequalities among the oldest old.** *Journal of Aging and Health, 6,* 51-69.

Describes the interaction of age and social class inequalities in health status for nationally representative sample of 537 elders age 77-98 from Sweden. Finds clear social class differences in health in this age group, and these inequalities are found both for men and women. The prevalence of illnesses and self-rated poor health among men who are farmers and self-employed, unskilled workers, or skilled workers is twice that of men who formerly are nonmanual works and professionals. [2.1, 2.4]

<144> Verbrugge, L. M. (1989). **The twain meet: Empirical explanations of sex differences in health and mortality.** *Journal of Health and Social Behavior, 30,* 282-304.

Identifies reasons for men's better health, using data from the Health in Detroit Study. Three kinds of risk factors are considered--acquired risks, psychosocial risks, and health-reporting behavior. Men's morbidity is influenced by social factors--risks stemming for employment, lower felt stress and unhappiness, and lessor feelings of vulnerability to illness. When all of the risk factors are controlled, the gender gap in morbidity narrows considerably. Indicators of chronic conditions and general health reverse to reveal higher morbidity for men, and men reveal greater disability and medical care. Men's disadvantage in health seems to have a biological basis. [2.1]

<145> Young, R. F., & Kahana, E. (1993). **Gender, recovery from late life heart attack, and medical care.** *Women and Health, 20,* 11-31.

Explores the recovery patterns for 162 men and 84 women age 43-87 in the aftermath of myocardial infarction. Analysis show the male MI patients are less likely to die during the first year and have more chance of full recovery. Cardiac symptoms decline for the men, and it appears that men receive more opportunities for state-of-the-art medical and surgical management of their heart conditions. Although the men are younger than the women, an interaction term considering age and gender does not predict mortality. Rather, social, medical, and demographic factors are implicated in the lessor risk of death and reinfarction shown by men. [2.1, 2.5]

<146> Zick, C. D., & Smith, K. R. (1991). **Marital transitions, poverty, and gender differences in mortality.** *Journal of Marriage and the Family, 53,* 327-336.

Examines what affect recent marital transitions v. changes in economic status have in explaining marriage-related mortality differentials. As prior studies suggest, there is a protective effect of marriage, and this protective effect is partly economic in nature for men and very much so for women. The social environment decreases men's, but not women's risks of mortality. As personal tastes or through social pressures, married men engage in less risky health-related behaviors (e.g., smoking, heavy drinking), and they have the support of wives. Not only marital status, but the transition from married to divorced, appears to increase the risk of dying for men. [2.1, 10.1]

SUCCESSFUL AGING

<147> Aldwin, C. M., Spiro, A. 3rd, Levenson, M. R., & Bosse, R.   (1989). Longitudinal findings from the Normative Aging Study: I. Does mental health change with age. *Psychology and Aging, 4,* **295-306.**

Investigates changes in self-reported symptoms using the Cornell Medical Index in a sample of 2,041 men who completed the CMI two or more times. Regressing symptoms against time, the slope of physical symptoms has a moderate increase over time and the slope of psychological symptoms indicates little change. Age accounts for 50 percent of the variance in physical symptoms when individual differences in change are examined, but age can not explain psychological symptoms.   A U-shaped curve describes the relation between age and psychological symptom change. [2.2, 2.3]

<148> Bolla-Wilson, K., & Bleecker, M. L. (1989).   Absence of depression in elderly adults. *Journals of Gerontology: Psychological Sciences, 44,* **P53-P55.**

Examines the effects of age and gender on the Beck Depression Inventory, the MMPI Scale 2, and Geriatric Depression Scale. No age effects are found on any of the depression scales' total scores. More somatic complaints are reported by the older group on the BDI, and fewer depressed items are reported by men on the MMPI-2. The findings underscore how the increased prevalence of somatic complaints are misinterpreted as representing more depression. [2.2]

<149> Blumenthal, J. A., Emery, C. F., Madden, D. J., Schniebolk, S., Walsh-Riddle, M., George, L. K., McKee, D. C., Higginbotham, M. B., Cobb, F. R., & Coleman, R. E. (1991). Long-term effects of exercise on psychological functioning in older men and women. *Journals of Gerontology: Psychological Sciences, 46,* **P352-P361.**

Determines the psychological, behavioral, and cognitive changes associated with up to 14 months of aerobic exercise training. For the first 4 months of the study, older men and women (N = 101) were assigned to one of three conditions--aerobic exercise, Yoga, or a waiting list control group. Men in the aerobic group became less depressed. A semi-crossover design stipulated that, following completion of the second assessment, all subjects completed 4 months of aerobic exercise and a third assessment of mood and cognitive functioning. Gender differences are observed in neuropsychological test performance--men achieve more taps than women. [2.2, 2.5]

<150> Girzadas, P. M., Counte, M. A., Glandon, G. L., & Tancredi, D. (1993). An analysis of elderly health and life satisfaction. *Behavior, Health, and Aging, 3,* **103-117.**

Explores the relationship between personal life satisfaction and health status among older persons. The model includes attributes that might moderate health status-life satisfaction. Logistic regressions find a consistently positive relationship between measures of men's life satisfaction and health status (functional and self-assessed). None of the personal attributes (e.g., martial status, socioeconomic status, health locus of control) provide enough additional information to contribute to the model. Functional health status is the strongest predictor. Findings are discussed in connection with some implications of health-related quality of life interventions. [2.2, 2.3]

<151> **Habte-Gabr, E., Wallace, R. B., Colsher, P. L., Hulbert, J. R., White, L. R., & Smith, I. M. (1991). Sleep patterns in rural elders: Demographic, health, and psychobehavioral correlates.** *Journal of Clinical Epidemiology, 44,* 5-13.

Occurring with increasing age are altered sleep patterns, including changes in bedtime, sleep latency, total sleep time, and arising time. Examines self-reported patterns for 3097 rural elders. Hours of sleep increase with age, with older respondents going to bed earlier; yet, reports of feeling rested in the morning decrease with age. Men go to bed later, have more hours of sleep, and are more likely to report feeling rested than women. Sleep patterns are related to health status, physical status, alcohol use, depressive symptomalogy, and social and recreational activity, and sleep problems are often associated with treatable health conditions. [2.2]

<152> **Hale, W. D., & Cochran, C. D. (1988). Gender differences in health attitudes among the elderly.** *Clinical Gerontologist, 4* (3), 23-27.

Investigates how gender affects the relationship between physical illness and levels of anxiety, depression, and other forms of psychological distress. Finds in in-depth data on 29 elderly men and 23 women that for men, not women, self-ratings of health and anxiety are correlated. Men have greater anxiety about death and more psychologically dysfunctional beliefs about illness and physical decline Concludes that physical decline of aging has a more pronounced psychological effect on men. [2.2, 2.5]

<153> **Haug, M. R., Breslau, N., & Folmar, S. J. (1989). Coping resources and selective survival in mental health of the elderly.** *Research on Aging, 11,* 468-491.

Demonstrates with longitudinal data (1975-1984) that poorer self-assessed physical health and social support emerge as resources for forestalling decline in mental health over a nine-year period. However, these resources have no effect in loss of cognitive ability, which suggests a biological component in this loss. Mortality over the nine-year time span is related to poorer initial mental health and cognitive ability, which demonstrates how survival masks the extent to which mental conditions decline over time. Impaired white men are the least likely to survive. Warns how measures of mental health and cognitive skills play a role in predicting mortality, but are less significant in explanatory power than the availability of social resources. [2.2, 7.5]

<154> **Hooker, K., & Siegler, I. C. (1993). Life goals, satisfaction, and self-rated health: Preliminary findings.** *Experimental Aging Research, 19,* 97-110.

Examines 203 elders' life goals, satisfaction, and self-rated health. Data from the Duke Second Longitudinal Study demonstrate that, on average, participants feel that they achieve most of their goals in the domains of family and interpersonal relationships, which both men and women identify as the most important domains. Most do not assess their interpersonal goals as "all achieved," because they anticipate further gains in these areas. Oldest respondents rate their achievements more highly, which may mean people eventually meet their goals in the interpersonal and family domains or adjust their perceptions so they are satisfied with their accomplishments. Perceived importance of goals explains a significant portion of differences in health, but not satisfaction. Goal achievement is predictive of both. [1.2, 2.2]

<155> Kastenbaum, R. (1994). Saints, sages, and sons of bitches: Three models for the grand old man. *Journal of Geriatric Psychiatry, 27*, 61-78.

Reviews three models of successful aging for men which have survived generations--the Saint, the Sage, and the Son of a Bitch (SOB). Each model reveals a partial truth about the meaning of advanced age. The Saint lives a pious life few emulate and represents the heroism of an ardent spirit that copes with a failing body in an imperfect world. The SOB seldom receives official acclaim as a model for successful aging, but the SOB wins sneaking admiration for being unrepentant, unadjusted, and unmoved by social expectations. He represents the heroism of an ardent spirit that copes with a failing body and an imperfect world. The Sage or wise old man is honored at the expense of being denied full personhood. He is the observer who is condemned to finding coherence, justice, truth, and beauty in the world. It is argued that men are no longer required to settle for these models. New models for the "grand old man" are not only a possibility but a necessity. [2.2, 6.2]

<156> Kessler, R. C., Foster, C., Webster, P. S., & House, J. S. (1992). The relationship between age and depressive symptoms in two national surveys. *Psychology and Aging, 7*, 119-126.

Reviews an inconsistency in the relationship between age and self-reported depressive symptoms. Most studies use screening scales that contain somatic items which can introduce an age bias. As important, most studies combine samples of men and women even though there is evidence that the sex difference in depressive symptoms varies by age. Addresses both these issues, using data from two large surveys (Americans' Changing Lives and National Survey of Families and Households). There are consistent, quite modest nonlinear associations between age and somatic symptoms and age and nonsomatic depressive affect in both surveys. Unlike prior evidence showing sex differences by age, with psychological distress more different for men and women in mid-life than early adulthood or old age, the authors found no significant gender difference in the age curves. [2.2, 2.3]

<157> Lewinsohn, P. M., Rohde, P., Seeley, J. R., & Fischer, S. A. (1991). Age and depression: Unique and shared effects. *Psychology & Aging, 6*, 247-260.

Tries to distinguish the concomitants of depression from the concomitants of aging, and examines the extent to which psychosocial variables associated with depression are also associated with age in three samples of 4,617 community residents age 50 and older. With few exceptions, age is not correlated with depression-related psychosocial variables. Rather, age is most associated with levels in neuropsychological and psychophysiological functioning. Several gender differences arose. For women more than men, older age is strongly associated with reduced self-esteem and lowered social support. For men, old age is associated with reductions in activity level. Further, the concomitants of depression in men and women differ in important ways. [2.2]

<158> Linsk, N. L. (1994). HIV and the elderly. *Families in Society, 75,* 362-372.

Discusses the substantial and increasing number of people who develop HIV infections in their later years. Most are associated with men's homosexual contact or blood transfusions. The author urges human service practitioners to become sensitive to the needs of HIV affected elders and their families. Discusses the value of prevention as part of initial engagement and assessment of elder persons. [2.2, 12.2]

<159> McDaniel, S. A., & McKinnon, A. L. (1993). Gender differences in informal support and coping among elders: Findings from Canada's 1985 and 1990 General Social Surveys. *Journal of Women and Aging, 5,* 79-98.

Uses data from Canada's 1985 General Social Survey on Health and Social Support and 1990 General Social Survey on Family and Friends, and examines elders' health status and ties with family and friends. Finds activity limitations due to a physical, mental, or chronic health condition increase with age less for men than women. Gender differences in longevity have important implications for coping and informal support in later life. Men are more likely to live until death as part of an intact marriage in which they receive emotional support and informal care from their spouse. In this study, men in poor health also have the least frequent contact with others, whereas women in poor health have the most frequent. [2.2, 7.5]

<160> McIntosh, W. A., Kaplan, H. B., Kubena, K. S., & Landmann, W. A. (1993). Life events, social support, and immune response in elderly individuals. *International Journal of Aging and Human Development, 37,* 23-36.

Investigates the effects of recent life events and social support on immune response. Regression analyses run separately for men (and women) indicate that differing aspects of social support have a direct positive impact on immune response for elderly men but had no mediating or buffering effects. Recent sexual dysfunction lowers lymphocyte count, while psychological adjustment and percentage kin in the intimate network elevated it. [2.2, 6.2, 7.5]

<161> Mishra, S. I., Aldwin, C. M., Colby, B. N., & Oseas, R. S. (1991). Adaptive potential, stress, and natural killer cell activity in older adults. *Journal of Aging and Health, 3,* 368-385.

Examines the relationship among psychosocial vulnerability and resilience and measures of self-reported physical symptoms, positive and negative affect, and natural killer cell activity in 39 men and women residing in a retirement community. Findings show that life events are directly related to physical health symptoms, and perceived stress and adaptive potential are associated with positive and negative affect. There is a tendency for adaptive potential to buffer the effect of perceived stress on negative affect. Natural killer cell activity is not significantly related to any psychosocial vulnerability and resilience factors. [2.1, 2.2]

<162> Mitteness, L. S. (1987). The management of urinary incontinence by community-living elderly. *The Gerontologist, 27,* 185-192.

Reports the ways elder people manage urinary incontinence and the reasons they make little use of health professionals. As part of a broader ethnographic study of the management of chronic illness, thirty incontinent elderly persons living in subsidized housing for seniors reveal that they routinely dismiss their urinary incontinence as a normal part of aging and use behavioral and psychological coping strategies to maintain their independence. Strategies evolve around keeping a discreditable condition invisible and protecting self-esteem. Men rely upon urine collecting devices (pads), and more than women they rely on treatment by a physician. Men's strategies also tend toward passively accepting or denying the existence of their bladder control problems. [2.2]

<163> **Mobily, P. R., Herr, K. A., Clark, M. K., & Wallace, R. B. (1994). An epidemiologic analysis of pain in the elderly: The Iowa 65+ Rural Health Study.** *Journal of Aging and Health, 6,* 139-154.

Reports a study of the prevalence and nature of pain in a population of 3,097 rural persons 65 years and older. Logistic regression analysis finds no significant association between the prevalence of overall pain and either gender or age. Roughly 86 percent of the older men and women report pain of some type in the year prior to the interview, and nearly 60 percent report multiple pain complaints. Joint pain is the most prevalent site reported. Men are much less likely than women to report back pain. Concludes that pain is a symptom of clinical importance, is prevalent among elders, and requires clinical management, not normalization. [2.2, 12.2]

<164> **Murrell, S. A., & Himmelfarb, S. (1989). Effects of attachment bereavement and pre-event conditions on subsequent depressive symptoms in older adults.** *Psychology and Aging, 4,* 166-172.

Recognizes that the loss of a valued person is a common clinical hypothesis in the an etiology of depression. Interviews a sample of 1,411 older adults age 55 and older both prior to and after bereavement. Men and women who lost a parent, spouse, or child equally show a steep increase in depression, higher levels of depression within the immediate 6-month interval following death, and an almost equally steep decrease within a year. [2.2]

<165> **Pavalko, E. K., Elder, G. H., & Clipp, E. C. (1993). Worklives and longevity: Insights from a life course perspective.** *Journal of Health and Social Behavior, 34,* 363-380.

In keeping with research on how work stress influences health or mortality, explores the implications of different patterns of career mobility on middle-class men's longevity. Tracking men's career pathways with the life history data in the Stanford-Terman study shows the pattern and order of jobs can lengthen or shorten men's lives. Few men experience a period in which they move through a series of unrelated jobs, but those who do have higher mortality risk. Similarly, men who progress early in their careers but then remain stable in later periods tend to be at a greater risk. Lowest risk is among men who progress in both time periods. Concludes that well-being is shaped by not just the advantageous and disadvantageous conditions of work, but the pattern and order of jobs. [2.2]

<166> Quam, J. K., & Whitford, G. S. (1992). Adaptation and age-related expecta-
tions of older gay and lesbian adults. *The Gerontologist, 32,* 367-374.

Summarizes a study of Midwestern lesbian women (N = 39) and gay men (N = 41) age
50 and older who have high involvement in the gay community. More men in the
sample live alone and are not involved in a relationship. The group reports acceptance
of the aging process and high levels of life satisfaction, despite problems associated
with both aging and sexual orientation. Those over 60 participate in religious activities
less than the under age 60. Asked to discuss problems specific to aging as a lesbian or
gay man, no single issue emerges as clearly as health, although men report fewer
health and income problems. Concludes being active in the gay community assists
acceptance of aging, because the gay community is accepting and the stress of being a
sexual minority enhances psychological and spiritual dimensions of life. [2.2, 2.3]

<167> Roos, N. P., & Havens, B. (1991). Predictors of successful aging: A twelve-
year study of Manitoba elderly. *American Journal of Public Health, 81,* 63-
68.

To study "successful aging," a representative cohort of Canadian elders age 65 to 84 (N
= 3,573) are interviewed in 1971 and the survivors of this cohort reinterviewed in 1983.
More than 100 indicators of demographic and socioeconomic status, social supports,
health and mental status in 1971, morbidity and access to health care during 1971-82,
are available to whether or not an individual lives to an advanced age, continues to
function well at home, and remains mentally alert. Those who age successfully are
shown to have greater satisfaction with life in 1983 and to have made fewer demands
on the health care system than those who aged less well. Regardless of the number of
potential predictors, only age, four measures of health status, two measures of mental
status, and not having one's spouse die or enter a nursing home are predictive of
successful aging. [2.2]

<168> Seeman, T. E., Rodin, J., & Albert, M. (1993). Self-efficacy and cognitive
performance in high-functioning older individuals: MacArthur studies of
successful aging. *Journal of Aging and Health, 5,* 455-474.

Examines the hypothesis that stronger self-efficacy beliefs are associated with better
cognitive performance at older ages. The sample of 531 men and 661 women age 70-
79 shows instrumental efficacy beliefs are related to better performance on tests of
memory and abstraction, independent of sociodemographic characteristics and
measures of physical and psychological health. For men, instrumental efficacy beliefs
have significant associations with cognitive ability, yet no association with cognitive
performance. [1.3, 2.2]

<169> Strawbridge, W. J., Camacho, T. C., Cohen, R. D., & Kaplan, G. A. (1993).
Gender differences in factors associated with change in physical function
in older age: A 6-year longitudinal study. *The Gerontologist, 33,* 603-609.

Theorizes that physical functioning underlies an older person's ability to remain
independent and active. Compares 147 men and 209 women age 65-95 who are part of
the initial cohort of the Alameda County Study to determine change in their functioning
across 6 years. Greater income and education and remaining married have significantly

strong associations with maintaining a positive functional status for men, and men who exercise and do not smoke also benefit. Gender-specific models are necessary to understand and determine older men's well-being. [2.2, 2.3, 2.5]

<170> Vaillant, G. E. (1990). Avoiding negative life outcomes: Evidence from a forty-five year study. In P. B. Baltes and M. M. Baltes (Eds.), *Successful aging: Perspectives from the behavioral sciences.* New York: Cambridge University Press.

Predictors of successful aging are examined among a sample of 204 older men who have been follow from when they were sophomores in 1940, 1941, and 1943 at Harvard University. Mental health between the ages of 30 and 50 is the best predictor of health outcomes in later life. Many potential variables that are important in adolescence and young adulthood are not predictive of older adults' adjustment. The most important variables in causing shifts from good to poor psychosocial adjustment are the onset of poor physical health or alcoholism. Personal qualities of perseverance and self-control assume greater importance in later life. Earlier stoicism and self discipline also become important. [1.3, 2.2]

<171> Vaillant, G. E. (1991). The association of ancestral longevity with successful aging. *Journals of Gerontology: Psychological Sciences, 46,* P292-P298.

Follows a cohort of 184 men (the Grant Study) from socioeconomically advantaged ancestors to age 65 to test the hypothesis that ancestral longevity predicts both mental and physical well-being. Findings indicate that ancestral longevity is strongly predictive of men's chronic illness at age 60 and mortality at age 68. Long-lived ancestors, however, do not effect psychosocial vigor or mental health at age 65. [2.2]

<172> Vaillant, G. E., & Vaillant, C. O. (1990). Natural history of male psychological health, XII: A 45-year study of predictors of successful aging at age 65. *American Journal of Psychiatry, 147,* 31-37.

Examines the lives of 173 white men prospectively from ages 18 to 65 to determine predictors of psychosocial and physical vitality in later life. Data are the longitudinal Grant Study of Harvard men in the early 1940s. Biopsychosocial predictors, gathered before age 50, are correlated with three outcomes at age 65: physical health, mental health, and life satisfaction. Finds several characteristics of major etiologic importance: long-lived ancestors, sustained familial relationships, absence of alcoholism, and absence of depressive disorder. Extent of tranquilizer use before age 50 is the most powerful negative predictor of both mental and physical health. [2.2]

PSYCHOLOGICAL WELL-BEING

<173> Adelman, M. (1990). Stigma, gay lifestyles, and adjustment to aging: A study of later-life gay men and lesbians. *Journal of Homosexuality, 20* (3-4), 7-32.

Examines adjustment to late life in terms of developmental, personal, and social styles of being gay using interviews with 27 older gay men and 25 older lesbians. Adjustment to aging is related to the particular style of being gay, satisfaction with being gay, and the developmental sequence of early gay events, and adjustment is related to high life satisfaction, low self-criticism, and few psychosomatic problems. Gay men meet the same developmental challenges as heterosexuals, and the only unique developmental aspect is the exacerbating influence of stigma on the maturational process. [1.1, 2.3]

<175> Aldwin, C. M., Levenson, M. R., & Spiro, A. 3rd. (1994). **Vulnerability and resilience to combat exposure: Can stress have lifelong effects?** *Psychology and Aging, 9,* 34-44.

Examines whether appraisals of desirable and undesirable effects of military service mediate the effects of combat stress on posttraumatic stress disorder symptoms in later life among 1,287 veterans age 44-91. The men report more desirable effects of military service (e.g., coping skills, competence, self-esteem) than undesirable ones, and both increase linearly with combat exposure. Perceived undesirable effects of service increase the effects of combat exposure on symptoms, and desirable events decrease effects of combat exposure on symptoms, even after controlling for depression and coping style. [2.3, 4.4]

<175> Ames, A., & Molinari, V. (1994). **Prevalence of personality disorders in community-living elderly.** *Journal of Geriatric Psychiatry and Neurology, 7,* 189-194.

Studies the prevalence of personality disorders in 100 older men and 100 older women which are anchored to DSM-III-R criteria. Results indicate a tendency toward fewer personality disorders in older than younger adults. Older women with personality disorders outnumber the older men slightly but nonsignificantly with disorders, and there are fewer prior consultations with a mental health professional for older men. [1.3, 2.3]

<176> Andersson, L., & Stevens, N. (1993). **Associations between early experiences with parents and well-being in old age.** *Journals of Gerontology: Psychological Sciences, 48,* P109-P116.

Explores the well-being and the impact of early experiences with parents on well-being in old age for 267 elderly community residents age 65-74 in Stockholm. Finds men demonstrate fewer psychosomatic symptoms, better subjective health, higher self-esteem, and lower anxiety and depression than women. But men are lonelier. Warm and attentive early experiences with parents does have a positive impact for men, and this effect of paternal and maternal care is stronger for unmarried older men. [1.3, 2.3]

<177> Angel, J. L., & Angel, R. J. (1992). **Age at migration, social connections, and well-being among elderly Hispanics.** *Journal of Aging and Health, 4,* 480-499.

Examines the effects of life course stage at migration and acquired social contacts on self-assessed health, functional disability, and life satisfaction for elderly Cuban Americans, Mexican Americans, and Puerto Ricans in the United States. Data are the

1988 National Survey of Hispanic Elderly People. Immigration late in life very likely undermines emotional well-being and interferes with the ability to perform basic activities in daily living, but significantly less so for men. Older Cuban Americans report consistently better health, less disability, and greater life satisfaction than other Latinos, and they seem to benefit from living in ethnic enclaves in which they have largely duplicated their culture of origin. [2.3, 11.2]

<178> Arens, D. A. (1982-83). Widowhood and well-being: An examination of sex differences within a causal model. *International Journal of Aging and Human Development, 15,* 27-40.

Explores the effects of widowhood on social participation and well-being for 579 men and 952 women age 65 and older. Data are from the 1974 National Council on Aging. Hypothesizes that widowhood has an adverse impact on well-being, especially among men. Finds an overall decline in well-being among the widowed, and men do not suffer a greater decline. The direct effects of widowhood are seldom substantial after factors such as health, socioeconomic status, and levels of social participation are taken into account. Poor health and low, fixed economic resources decrease feelings of well-being. Contrary to expectation, widowed men do not show a consistent pattern of reduced social participation. [2.3, 10.1]

<179> Arfken, C. L., Lach, H. W., Birge, S. J., & Miller, J. P. (1994). The prevalence and correlates of fear of falling in elderly persons living in the community. *American Journal of Public Health, 84,* 565-570.

Examines the prevalence of fear of falling and its association with measures of falling, quality of life, and frailty among 1,358 adults age 65 and older from St. Louis. The prevalence of fear increases with age and is smaller in men. After gender and age adjustments, those who are fearful of falling have an elevated risk for worse quality of life--decreased satisfaction with life, increased frailty and depressed mood, and recent experience with falls. [2.3]

<180> Blazer, D., Burchett, B., Service, C., & George, L. K. (1991). The association of age and depression among the elderly: An epidemiologic exploration. *Journals of Gerontology: Medical Sciences, 46,* M210-M215.

Recognizes that advanced age is hypothesized to be a risk factor for depression, yet studies do not uniformly support this hypothesis. The Duke EPESE (Establishment of a Population for Epidemiologic Studies of the Elderly) assessed 3,998 community-dwelling elders age 65 and older for depressive symptoms, using a modified version of the CES-D. Finds depressive symptoms in bivariate analysis associated with women, increased age, lower income, physical disability, cognitive impairment, and lack of social support. The association of age and depressive symptoms reverses when the confounding variables are controlled in regression analyses. Concludes oldest old suffered fewer depressive symptoms. [2.2, 2.3]

<181> Bosse, R., Aldwin, C. M., Levenson, M. R., & Ekerdt, D. J. (1987). Mental health differences among retirees and workers: Findings from the Normative Aging Study. *Psychology and Aging, 2,* 383-389.

Reviews findings which show little effect of retirement on physical health, and unclear effects on mental health. Examines psychological symptoms in a sample of 1,513 older men, and finds that retirees reported more symptoms than did workers, even after controlling for physical health status. Analyses examining the circumstances of retirement find no effects for length of retirement or part-time employment, but for the timing of retirement. Both early and late retirees report more symptoms, particularly somatization--the frequency of relatively minor, nonspecific aches and pains. [2.3, 10.2]

<182> Brabant, S., Forsyth, C. J., & Melancon, C. (1992). Grieving men: Thoughts, feelings, and behaviors following the deaths of wives. *Hospice Journal, 8,* 33-47.

Comments on how little attention has been given to the impact of bereavement on men. Explores the thoughts, feelings, and behaviors of twenty men following the deaths of their wives. Findings do not support prevailing assumptions that men are less likely to be emotionally involved in the conjugal relationship and, thus, less likely to grieve than women. Concludes that death of a wife may evoke intense feelings. The majority of men knew they hurt, but they did not reach out to others for help. [2.3]

<183> Brown, D. R., Milburn, N. G., & Gary, L. E. (1992). Symptoms of depression among older African-Americans: An analysis of gender differences. *The Gerontologist, 32,* 789-795.

Investigates the association between gender and depressive symptoms in a community-based sample of 148 African-Americans age 65 and older. Finds no gender difference in overall level of depressive symptomatology. Further analyses suggest that the lack of a gender difference in depressive symptoms is attributable to similarities in risk factors related to stressful life events and the social roles associated with employment and child rearing. [2.3]

<184> Burton, R. P., Rushing, B., Ritter, C., & Rakocy, A. (1993). Roles, race and subjective well-being: A longitudinal analysis of elderly men. *Social Indicators Research, 28,* 137-156.

Examines the impact of race and social roles on subjective well-being in elderly men, using data from the National Longitudinal Survey of Labor Market Experience. Data are interviews with 2,285 men age 55-69 at Time 1 and 60-74 years at Time 2. Contrary to expectations, results do not indicate lower subjective well-being for black men than for white men. Findings demonstrate that particular role configurations affect happiness and that these effects are different for blacks and whites. [2.3]

<185> Callahan, C. M., & Wolinsky, F. D. (1994). The effect of gender and race on the measurement properties of the CES-D in older adults. *Medical Care, 32,* 341-356.

Investigates the extent to which known differences in the prevalence of symptoms of depression among older adults in four race-gender groups are explained by the properties of the CES-D scale. At face value, it would appear that black men have the fewest symptoms, and white men are between black and white women. Finds the actual experience versus expression of depressive symptoms may vary too significantly. The differential response tendencies vary too socioculturally by age, race, and gender to compare rates of depressive symptoms. [2.3]

<186> Charmaz, K. (1994). Identity dilemmas of chronically ill men. *Sociological Quarterly, 35,* 269-288.

Chronic illness frequently comes to men suddenly with immediate intensity, severity, and uncertainty, and men's responses are personal gender constructions. Explores how men experience chronic illness and how assumptions about masculinity affect men's identity dilemmas and "masculinizing practices." Using qualitative data (40 depth inter-views of 20 men), examines the processes of awakening to denigrated or shameful identities after a life-threatening crisis, accommodating to uncertainty as the men realize that illness onset has lasting consequences, and preserving self amidst the experience of loss and change. Finds that illness marginalizes men's sense of masculinity and control, physical dependence is demeaning, and some men cast wives and physicians into the role of adversaries to maintain their status in the hierarchy of men. Traditional assumptions about male identity--the emphasis on personal autonomy and bravery--form a two-educed sword for men in chronic illness. [2.1, 2.3]

<187> Chatters, L. M. (1988). Subjective well-being evaluations among older black Americans. *Psychology and Aging, 3,* 184-190.

Investigates the relations among social status and resources, health and stress factors, and a single-item measure of subjective well-being (happiness) in a sample of 581 black adults age 55 and older. Discovers older black men and women are not different in expressed satisfaction with health, despite real differences in perceptions of disability. Discusses how older men appear to expect and tolerate less disability than do older women, which yields the no difference finding. The age and gender differences in health status suggest the elderly blacks may have normative expectations for health that are related to these statuses. [2.3]

<188> Chiriboga, D. A. (1982). Adaptation to marital separation in later and earlier life. *Journal of Gerontology, 37,* 109-114.

Psychosocial functioning is assessed in a sample of 310 men and women who recently separated from their spouses and range in age from 20 to 79. Results indicate men of all ages are less happy and exhibit less improvement in perceived health status from before to after separation. The findings also support the hypothesis that older people are more vulnerable to the process of divorce than are younger people. Older respondents are more unhappy and report fewer positive emotional experiences. They show more social discomfort and view both the past and the future with greater pessimism and long-term dissatisfaction. Many older respondents are unable to project even 1 year into the future. Older men appear most vulnerable in this respect. [2.3]

<189> Cicirelli, V. C. (1989). Feelings of attachment to siblings and well-being in later life. *Psychology and Aging, 4,* 211-216.

Hypothesizes that the well-being of older persons depends on their perception of the closeness of the sibling bond, disruptions to the bond, and the sex combination of the siblings. Interviews 83 people age 61 to 91, and presents separate correctional analyses on the four sex combinations of siblings. The closeness of the bond to a sister was related to less depression for both men and women. Because the age cohorts interviewed were reared at a time when very traditional sex role conditioning was the norm, and when women were expected to maintain closer family ties and assume caregiving activities, concludes that these same cultural expectations make it upsetting to lose a sister's support. [2.3, 8.1]

<190> Clayton, P. J. (1979). Sequelae and nonsequelae of conjugal bereavement. *American Journal of Psychiatry, 136,* 1530-1534.

Reviews prospective studies of morbidity and mortality following the death of a spouse. Finds few changes in older men's and women's physical health, visits to physicians, and number of hospitalizations. By contrast, the bereaved report significant depressive symptoms during the first year, but psychiatric consultation is rare, and psychiatric hospitalization is so infrequent that bereavement need not be considered a cause of mental illness. Although studies yield conflicting results, there may be greater mortality for men, especially older men, during the first six months of bereavement. Unreplicated is an increase in suicides during the first four years of bereavement, most of which was accounted for by men aged 60 or over during the first year. [2.3, 4.1]

<191> Cohen-Sachs, B. (1993). Coping with the stress of aging--creatively. *Stress Medicine, 9,* 45-49.

Summarizes a conference presentation on creatively coping with the stresses of aging, and theorizes the "best youth elixir" can be found in two words--keep moving. The person who ages successfully is perceived to be one who finds new activities to replace those that he or she outgrows or is forced to give up. Elders are advised to keep challenging themselves to maintain their intellectual acuity. Continued activity can be a "tonic" for boredom and frustration that can lead to immune system disorders, and a good laugh acts as a "mini work-out" to stimulate the cardiovascular, respiratory, and nervous systems. [1.3, 2.3]

<192> Coke, M. M. (1992). Correlates of life satisfaction among elderly African Americans. *Journals of Gerontology: Psychological Sciences, 47,* P316-P320.

Although previous studies show life satisfaction is correlated with perceived health and adequacy of income, African-Americans are typically poorer and less healthy than older whites, which suggests other factors contribute to life satisfaction. Examines correlates of older African Americans' life satisfaction (87 males and 79 females). Finds among men, family role involvement and hours of church participation are significantly related to life satisfaction, as is self-perceived adequacy of income, actual household income, educational level, and self-rated religiosity. [2.3, 5.1]

<193> Connidis, I. A., & McMullin, J. A. (1993). To have or have not: Parent status and the subjective well-being of older men and women. *The Gerontologist, 33,* 630-636.

Calculates the effect of parent status on subjective well-being, as measured by avowed happiness, depression, and satisfaction with life. Finds considerable uniformity by gender. Close fathers and mothers report greater well-being than either distant parents or adults childless by circumstance, but no greater well-being that the adults childless by choice. Unlike the women, older men childless by circumstance are less happy than older fathers close to their children, and divorced men are less happy and more depressed than married men. [2.3, 8.2]

<194> Cryns, A. G., Gorey, K. M., & Goldstein, M. Z. (1990). Effects of surgery on the mental status of older persons: A meta-analytic review. *Journal of Geriatric Psychiatric and Neurology, 3,* 184-191.

Analyzes 18 empirical studies to determine the psychological effects of surgery on adults age 65 and older. Surgery has a significant, decompensating impact on the mental status of older persons, but less for men than women. Gender also seems to predict which kind of postsurgical impairment occurs, when impairment occurs. Men manifest less delirious symptomalogy but more cognitive decompensation. Findings affirm that age, then gender predict postoperative mental status. [2.3]

<195> Dean, A., Kolody, B., Wood, P., & Matt, G. E. (1992). The influence of living alone on depression in elderly persons. *Journal of Aging and Health, 4,* 3-18.

Distinguishes the affects of living alone on depressive symptoms from the influence of other highly relevant variables (social support, age, marital status) in a community sample of adults age 50 and older. Elderly persons who live alone have higher levels of symptomalogy, and this relationship is independent of the influence of expressive support from friends, face-to-face interaction with friends, undesirable life events, disability, and financial strain. The depressive effect of living alone is greater on men than women. [2.3, 11.2]

<196> Elder, G. H., & Clipp, E. C. (1989). Combat experience and emotional health: Impairment and resilience in later life. *Journal of Personality, 57,* 311-341.

Explores the legacy of combat with a sample of 149 veterans from World War II and the Korean conflict. Archival data from the Stanford-Terman study are used to determine the subjective experience of combat that veterans maintain in later life. The research also examines how these recollections are linked to the severity of combat and to postwar adaptations. Veterans of heavy combat are at greater risk of emotional and behavior problems throughout the postwar years. Clinical ratings also show these men become more resilient and less helpless over time when compared with other men. [1.2, 2.3]

<197> Farberow, N. L., Gallagher-Thompson, D., Gilewski, M. J., & Thompson, L. W. (1992). Changes in grief and mental health of bereaved spouses of older suicides. *Journals of Gerontology: Psychological Sciences, 47,* P357-P366.

Compares longitudinally over a bereavement period of two and a half years the effects of suicide death on surviving older spouses (55 years and older) to the effects of natural death on spouse survivors and a married non-bereaved control group. Regardless of the mode of death, the loss of a spouse is a difficult psychological trauma. Men report less anxiety, tension, and apprehension than women, especially within the first six months, perhaps because gender-influenced suicide rates leave more suicide widows than widowers. After two and a half years, most gender differences disappear, and men and women report resumption of personal and social function despite continuing feelings of sadness and loss. [2.3, 4.1]

<198> Farnsworth, J., Pett, M. A., & Lund, D. A. (1989). Predictors of loss management and well-being in later life widowhood and divorce. *Journal of Family Issues, 10,* 101-121.

Examines how older men and women adapt to change in their martial status. Participants are 109 recently divorced, nonremarried men and women and 110 widowed age 50-69. Data are collected 6, 12, 18, or 24 months after the loss, using self-report items on income adequacy, marital happiness, management of loss, and health. Older men tend to experience less difficulty in adjusting to widowhood or divorce than women, perhaps because positive ratings of self-reported personal health consistently indicate more satisfactory adjustment. Time since loss, marital happiness, and self-esteem are additional predictors of adjustment for widowed respondents. Divorced respondents reveal greater anger-guilt-confusion than the widowed respondents. [2.3]

<199> Feinson, M. C. (1985). Aging and mental health: Distinguishing myth from reality. *Research on Aging, 7,* 155-174.

A prevailing belief about older adults is that they are more psychologically distressed and/or depressed than younger adults. Analysis of 18 earlier studies finds 10 that show no age effect on distress, and 8 that show young adults more distressed. Most prior work combines elders into a single category (e.g., 60+ or 65+) suggesting age distinctions among elders are less important than for young and middle-age adults. In an original study involving a sample of 313 community-based elders, gender does not distinguish the distressed elders in regression analyses of 5 different distress measures. [2.3, 6.2]

<200> Ferraro, K. F. (1992). Self and older-people referents in evaluating life problems. *Journals of Gerontology: Social Sciences, 47,* S105-S114.

Examines the severity of the perceived life problems common among "older people" and the cohort changes in such perceptions over the period of 1974-1981. People of all ages, including older adults, evaluate other's problems as being more substantial than the same problems when evaluated for self. Older people are less likely to report serious personal problems, and they feel the seriousness of problems among elders decreased over time. Older men are likely to report less seriousness of life problems than older women at both surveys, even after controlling for age differences. [2.2, 2.3, 6.2]

<201> Folkman, S., Lazarus, R. S., Pimley, S., & Novacek, J. (1987). Age differences in stress and coping processes. *Psychology and Aging, 2,* **171-184.**

Reviews how normative stress, coping patterns, and the ways in which these patterns might differ in older and younger people. Compares older (75 men and 86 women) and younger (75 men and 75 women) adults' experiences of daily hassles and strategies for coping with the hassles. Older adults experience fewer hassles in domains of finances, work, personal life, and family and friends. Older men report relatively fewer financial hassles. They experience more health hassles, and they report more hassles having to do with political and social issues (and news events) and fewer with family and friends. By contrast, the gender effects on coping are not robust. Finds no differences in the two traditionally masculine forms of coping--confrontive coping and planful problem-solving. Further, virtually no age by gender interaction is evident. Older people use more passive, intrapersonal emotion-focused forms of coping (distancing, acceptance of responsibility, and positive reappraisal), rather than the more active, interpersonal problem-focused coping (confrontive coping, seeking of social support, planful problem solving). Findings are consistent with a developmental interpretation for age, but do not support the view that men and women have different trajectories. [1.4, 2.3, 6.2]

<202> Fontana, A., & Rosenheck, R. (1994). Traumatic war stressors and psychiatric symptoms among World War II, Korean, and Vietnam War veterans. *Psychology and Aging, 9,* **27-33.**

Tests three hypotheses regarding older veterans' symptoms of war-related posttraumatic stress disorder and general psychiatric distress: Symptoms are more severe the more severe the traumatic exposure, symptoms are less severe the older the veteran's age, and symptom levels differ across sociocultural cohorts. Studying 5,138 veterans seeking treatment from VA outpatient teams, all hypothesis are supported, testifying to the generality of war experiences. Having been the target of killing and having participated in abusive violence are related to emotional distress. [2.3]

<203> Frey, D. E., Kelbley, T. J., Durham, L., & James, J. S. (1992). Enhancing the self-esteem of selected male nursing home residents. *The Gerontologist, 32,* **552-557.**

Hypothesizes that self-esteem can be an important ingredient for the quality of life of institutionalized older adults, and investigates treatment procedures for enhancing the self-esteem of older men who are nursing home residents. Twenty-one subjects were assigned randomly to either a control group meeting to discuss current news events or an experimental group receiving 12 weeks of counseling intervention. Self-esteem significantly increases for the experimental subjects but not before they experience an initial, significant decrease in feelings of self worth. The mid-treatment observation of the dependent variable is a vital factor in discovering the curvilinear relationship between time and self-evaluations. Concludes that continuing to learn about oneself, and the nurturing of the self over time, make an important contribution to the quality of life. [2.3, 12.2]

<204> Frischer, M., Ford, G, & Taylor, R.   (1991).   Life events and psychological well-being in old age. *Psychology and Health, 5,* 203-219.

Reports how little attention has been paid to the prevalence of life-events among the elderly. Drawing from a three-wave longitudinal study of community-based elderly in Aberdeen, Scotland, finds negative life events are highly prevalent among both survivors (N =349) and non-survivors (N =108). Men are less likely to report non-health events. LISREL-modeling of the survivors reveals those in a poor psychological state are more likely to report serious non-health events than health event. Yet it is the health events that undermined psychological well-being, even after prior psychological state is taken into account. [2.2, 2.3]

<205> George, L. K., Blazer, D. G., Hughes, D. C., & Fowler, N.   (1989).   Social support and the outcome of major depression. *British Journal of Psychiatry, 154,* 478-485.

Evaluates longitudinally social network size and subjective social support received by 150 adults initially diagnosed with major depression. The two periods from which data are available are the initial interviews when inpatients and follow-up interviews 6-32 months later. Network size and, especially, support are predictors of depressive symptoms at follow-up. This effect is stronger for men, which means that inadequate social support is a potent predictor of older men's levels of depression. [2.3, 7.5]

<206> Gerson, L. W., Jarjoura, D., & McCord, G.   (1987).   Factors related to impaired mental health in urban elderly. *Research on Aging, 9,* 356-371.

Begins by addressing how research does not consistently reveal what factors covary with mental health status among the aged. Examines correlates of three mental health measures (subjectively defined status, scaled from the OARS, and interviewer-rated) in a sample of 1,139 elders. Poorer physical health, functional ability (ADLs), and economic resources are consistently associated with poorer mental health. Married men show better mental health than those not married or married women, and social resources seem important for women's mental health but less so for men. The patterns reveal that gender interacts with other factors to effect mental health. [2.3]

<207> Hastrup, J. L., Baker, J. G., Kraemer, D. L., & Bornstein, R. F.   (1986).   Crying and depression among older adults. *The Gerontologist, 26,* 91-96.

Research on crying is in its early stages. With self-reports of crying episodes for two nonclinical samples of younger and older men and women, determines how to interpret an elder's report of crying. Finds a weak relationship between crying and depression among older adults. Men do cry less than women, and gender is unrelated to the causes of crying. Older men report crying significantly more than younger men. [1.3, 2.3]

<208> Herzog, A. R., Fultz, N. H., Brock, B. M. Brown, M. B., & Diokno, A. C.   (1988).   Urinary incontinence and psychological distress among older adults. *Psychology and Aging, 3,* 115-121.

Urinary incontinence is a fairly common health problem among older adults, and is commonly assumed to have detrimental effect on the daily lives of elders. Examines the relationship between incontinence and psychological distress in a sample of 747 women and 541 men age 60 and older who were community-dwelling. The effect on well-being is apparent when assessed through measures of distress. Among men, the effect is not statistically significant, and the bivariate relationship between incontinence and distress (depression, negative affect, low life satisfaction) is weak. These findings fail to support an hypothesis of severe, broad-based psychological effects of urinary incontinence, at most, it has a very mild effect. [2.1, 2.3]

<209> Hickson, J., Housley, W. F., & Boyle, C. (1988). **The relationship of locus of control, age, and sex to life satisfaction and death anxiety in older persons.** *International Journal of Aging and Human Development, 26, 191-199.*

Examines the internal-external locus of control concept in relation to life satisfaction and death anxiety among community-dwelling men (N = 37) and women (N = 85) age 61 and older. Men reported higher life satisfaction and lower death anxiety than women, and for men control orientation was correlated with life satisfaction. The importance of the perception of controlling events to life satisfaction is discussed. [1.3, 2.3]

<210> Holahan, C. K. (1988). **Relation of life goals at age 70 to activity participation and health and psychological well-being among Terman's gifted men and women.** *Psychology and Aging, 3, 286-291.*

Explores the relationship of life goals in aging to activity involvement, health, and well-being. Questionnaires completed by 681 participants in the Terman Study between age 65 and 75 in 1982 reveal three goal scales (autonomy, involvement, and achievement motivation) are related to subjective health, but one (autonomy) is not related to well-being. Life goals contribute to health and well-being, both directly and indirectly, through activity participation. In most cases the indirect effect of life goals on health and well-being accounts for more than half of the total effect. These findings suggest that the association between goals and functioning is expressed behaviorally in activity involvement, which is then related to health and well-being. [2.3, 2.4]

<211> Holahan, C. K., & Holahan, C. J. (1987). **Life stress, hassles, and self-efficacy in aging: A replication and extension.** *Journal of Applied Social Psychology, 17, 574-592.*

Investigates the possible causal connections among life stress, hassles, and self-efficacy to emotional and physical health outcomes. Data are from a small sample of 26 men and 26 women between the ages of 65 and 75. Frequency of daily hassles is the strongest predictor of physical and emotional health, showing significant relationships with depression and somatic complaints both concurrently and one-year later. Perceived self-efficacy in dealing with both hassles and life events is also significantly linked to current and subsequent depression. The older men report better well-being and health than the women, perhaps because of gender differences in types of hassles and perceptions of self-efficacy. [1.1, 2.3]

<212> Husaini, B. A., Moore, S. T., Castor, R. S., Neser, W., Whitten-Stovall, R., Linn, J. G., & Griffin, D. (1991). Social density, stressors, and depression: Gender differences among the black elderly. *Journals of Gerontology: Psychological Sciences, 46*, P236-P242.

Interviews from 600 black elderly community residents (age 55-85) are used to study how social density and stressors differentially interact for elderly men and women to affect depressive symptomatology. Regression analyses find chronic medical problems are the common predictors of depression among both genders. For men, 48 percent live alone, and none of the social support dimensions covary with depression. Older women show more depression as the number of events increase, as level of contact with relatives and friends decrease, and as levels of social attachment decrease. These relationships tend to be stronger for 59% of the women who live alone. [2.3, 7.5]

<213> Johnson, C. L, & Barer, B. M. (1993). Coping and sense of control among the oldest old: An exploratory analysis. *Journal of Aging Studies, 7*, 67-80.

Increasing evidence identifies the relationship between a personal sense of control and health grows stronger with age. Studies on two modes of adaptation among 150 individuals, 85 years and older. Physical and social losses are sustained by many elders this age, yet most are also able to sustain a sense of well-being. Two adaptive techniques are observed: Individuals redefine their optimal level of social integration and become content with a narrower, more constricted social world; and, time orientation changes from the future to the present. [2.2, 2.3]

<214> Keith, V. M. (1993). Gender, financial strain, and psychological distress among older adults. *Research on Aging, 15*, 123-147.

Presumes the effect of gender on distress is not direct but mediated. Investigates if differential exposure and differential vulnerability to chronic financial strain contribute to less distress for among older men. Examines the effects of marital status, a factor responsible for differential exposure, and the effects of control, a coping resource affecting differential vulnerability. Finds financial strain is equally distressful to older men and women primarily because it reduces their ability to maintain a sense of control. Older men are exposed to less financial stress, and their differential exposure results, in part, from their probability of being married. With men and women at unequal risks, aggregate gender differences in reported distress are substantial. [2.3, 10.1]

<215> Koenig, H. G., Kvale, J. N., & Ferrel, C. (1988). Religion and well-being in later life. *The Gerontologist, 28*, 18-28.

Frequency of religious behaviors and level of intrinsic religiosity are less central to older men's lives than women's. Religiosity is highly associated with morale for women, not for men. Only church attendance and church-related activities covary with men's morale. [2.3, 5.1]

<216> Krause, N. (1991). Stressful events and life satisfaction among elderly men and women. *Journals of Gerontology: Social Sciences, 46*, S84-S92.

Examines the interrelationships among global and domain-specific life-satisfaction (e.g., with health and finances) and stressful events (e.g., illness and financial loss). Two competing theoretical approaches guide the study. A "bottom-up" perspective suggests that individuals compartmentalize feelings about their lives and from judgments about specific areas of life. A "tops down" approach suggests that people's ongoing views about life in general result in domain specific assessments that are congruent with the overall view. Analyses support the "bottom-up" perspective--illness and financial loss tend to affect their respective domain-specific satisfactions but not global life satisfaction. Older men are more satisfied with their financial situation and their health, and they express more life satisfaction than the older women. [2.3, 10.1]

<217> Lasher, K. P., & Faulkender, P. J. (1993). Measurement of aging anxiety: Development of the Anxiety about Aging Scale. *International Journal of Aging and Human Development,* **37, 247-259.**

Proposes that aging anxiety is a separate construct, distinct from other measures of anxiety and from related constructs such as psychological well-being and attitudes toward aging. Develops a measure of aging anxiety which reliably assesses four dimensions--fear of old people, psychological concerns, physical appearance anxiety, and fear of losses. Men are significantly more anxious about aging than women, age does not appear to influence anxiety (although age did correlate with physical appearance anxiety), and there is no interaction between gender and age. [2.3]

<218> Lawrence, R. H., & Liang, J. Structural integration of the Affect Balance Scale and the Life Satisfaction Index A: Race, sex, and age differences. *Psychology and Aging,* **3, 375-384.**

Determines race, sex, and age differences in the factorial structure of Liang's model of subjective well-being, which integrates the Affect Balance Scale and the Life Satisfaction Index A. Data are from the 1974 National Council on Aging Survey. The structure of the items are analyzed for factorial invariance for white and black subsamples, men and women, and the young-old and the old-old. Race differences are found in factorial structure, but sex and age differences are not, meaning that comparisons between elderly men and women are entirely appropriate. [2.3]

<219> Lewis, G. R., & Ishii-Kuntz, M. (1987). Social interaction, loneliness, and emotional well-being among the elderly. *Research on Aging,* **9, 459-482.**

Assesses the effects of interaction with different types of role partners on the emotional well-being of elders, and the extent to which these effects are mediated by feelings of social integration (or loneliness). Working with data on 2,872 adults age 55 and older, finds feelings of loneliness are reduced, and morale increased by health and interaction with friends. Interaction with children and grandchildren has no effect. For older men, neighborhood interaction, friends, being married, and income all reduce feelings of loneliness; and, men who report not feeling lonely, more interaction with friends, and participation in voluntary associations and church have the highest morale. [2.3]

<220> Linn, B. S., Linn, M. W., & Jensen, J. (1983). Surgical stress in the healthy elderly. *Journal of the American Geriatrics Society,* **31, 544-548.**

Examines the relationship between preoperative anxiety and postoperative outcomes in healthy young and elderly men. Findings reveal that old and young men do not differ significantly before surgery. When the age groups are divided by preoperative anxiety and their postoperative outcomes are compared, an association emerges between anxiety, a high number of disability days, and the use of pain-relieving medications in each age group. Elderly men who suffer from preoperative anxiety have more disability days and complications. [2.3, 12.2]

<221> Lubben, J. E. (1988). **Gender differences in the relationship of widowhood and psychological well-being among low income elderly.** *Women & Health,* *14,* 161-189.

Examines the influence of widowhood on the psychological well-being of low income elders. A sample of Medi-Cal recipients (California) includes 57 widowers, 99 married men, 393 widows, and 78 married women. Finds health status and social network variables are the strongest predictors of life satisfaction, and once health and social network variables are controlled, both widows and widowers have lower psychological well-being than their married counterparts. Discusses the influence of widowhood on the psychological well-being and how close friendships appear to aggravate rather than to buffer stress among elderly men. Family rather than friends are more pivotal to men's well-being. Implications for clinical practice are discussed. [2.3, 10.1]

<222> Lund, D. A., Caserta, M S., & Dimond, M. F. (1986). **Gender differences through two years of bereavement among the elderly.** *The Gerontologist,* *26,* 314-320.

Highlights evidence that conjugal bereavement has numerous psychological and social effects associated with it. Compares the bereavement process of elderly widowers and widows in a two-year longitudinal study. Bereaved persons (N = 192) age 50-92 are assessed at six time periods following the spouse's death, and no significant gender effects in the bereavement process are noted. Rather the process is characterized more by similarities. This does not mean that men experience the death of a spouse in the same manner as women, but their adaptation is much the same. They improve gradually with time, experience emotional highs and lows concurrently and emotional confusion, and continue to experience feelings and adjustment difficulties to new roles two-years after the spouse's death. [2.3]

<223> Matt, G. E., & Dean, A. (1993). **Social support from friends and psychological distress among elder persons: Moderator effects of age.** *Journal of Health and Social Behavior,* *34,* 187-200.

Examines the relationships among gender, age, friend support, and psychological distress over 22-months for young-old adults age 50-70 and old-old adults age 71 and older. Finds that different causal processes operate for the two age groups--the effects of friend support on distress and distress on friend support are only visible in the oldest group. They receive less friend support at follow-up if they had previously experienced psychological distress, and they are more distressed at follow-up if they had receive little support earlier. The old-olds in general, and old-old men in particular, are especially vulnerable to psychological distress when losing friend support, and to lose friend support when experiencing psychological distress. [2.3, 7.5]

<224> McGhee, J. I. (1985). Effects of siblings on the life satisfaction of the rural elderly. *Journal of Marriage and the Family, 47,* 85-91.

Prior research suggests siblings contribute to elders' life satisfaction and well-being, but no work has established that more frequent interaction with siblings contributes higher morale or life satisfaction. With a sample of 231 rural elders, tests the hypothesis that geographic proximity of same-sex siblings exerts a positive influence on life satisfaction. Finds geographical proximity of cross-sex siblings and frequency of sibling interaction are not significantly related to life satisfaction for either older men or women. Regression analysis reveal that among men, availability of a brother is positively associated with life satisfaction, but the effect is negligible. Concludes that the effects of cross-sex siblings and sibling interaction on the life satisfaction are relatively minor. Results indicate a need to explore the meaning of sibling relations in old age more thoroughly. [2.3, 8.1]

<225> Moritz, D. J., Kasl, S. V., & Berkman, L. F. (1989). The health impact of living with a cognitively impaired elderly spouse: Depressive symptoms and social functioning. *Journals of Gerontology: Social Sciences, 44,* S17-S27.

Identifies the social and psychological consequences of living with a cognitively impaired spouse among 318 community-dwelling elders pairs. Wives' cognitive impairment is associated with husband's depressive symptomalogy, but not the reverse. Husband's ill-health is affected directly and mediated through the "loss" of a spouse-- wife's functional limitations and lack of support, his household responsibilities and lack of participation in social-leisure activities. [2.3, 9.1]

<226> Mui, A. C. (1993). Self-reported depressive symptoms among black and Hispanic frail elders: A sociocultural perspective. *Journal of Applied Gerontology, 12,* 170-187.

Examines the sources of depressive symptoms experienced by 1,272 black and 211 Hispanic frail elderly persons. Men in both groups express less depressive symptoms than women, and Hispanics report more depressive symptoms than blacks. For Hispanics, the unique predictor of depressive symptoms is few informal helpers, whereas for blacks the predictors are a higher level of impairment in instrumental activities of daily living, loss of a significant other, involuntary relocation, and fewer formal care providers. What commonly predicts both groups' symptomalogy are number of physical illnesses, poor perceived health, and less sense of control in life. [2.3, 2.4]

<227> Nacoste, D. R. B., & Wise, E. H. The relationship among negative life events, cognitions, and depression within three generations. *The Gerontologist, 31,* 397-403.

Investigates whether the influence of cognitive factors on depression is consistent among generations. Colleges students (N = 58), 57 same-sex parents (age 39-63), and

56 same-sex grandparents (age 62-83) complete measures of stressful life events, dysfunctional attitudes, and depression. Finds no gender differences on dysfunctional attitudes or negative life-events, but men score lower on covert negative self-statements (or automatic thoughts). Finds negative thoughts significantly predict depression in the parent group, and combine with negative life events in the grandparents. Results demonstrate the role of cognitions in depression may differ as a function of generation. [2.3]

<228> Norris, F. H., & Murrell, S. A. (1987). Older adult family stress and adaptation before and after bereavement. *Journal of Gerontology, 42*, 606-612.

Studies prospectively 63 older adults who experience the death of a spouse, parent, or child, and 387 who are not bereaved. Three interviews before and one after the death reveal bereavement itself does not affect health, but it does have a strong effect on psychological distress regardless of level of prebereavement stress. Findings affirm that grief is psychological work for men. The tasks of bereavement begin well before the death event in managing family stress, can affect health, and the impact likely comes before rather than after the death and as a result of greater family stress. [2.3]

<229> Okun, M. A., Melichar, J. F., & Hill, M. D. (1990). Negative daily events, positive and negative social ties, and psychological distress among older adults. *The Gerontologist, 30*, 193-199.

Examines the stress-buffering effect of positive social ties on psychological distress in a sample of 110 community-dwelling elders age 60-89. Consistent with a stress-buffering hypothesis, the effect of negative daily events on distress decreases as positive social ties increase. Contrary to the stress-amplifying hypothesis, negative social ties do not interact with negative events, rather they have an independent, additive effect. These patterns are not directly affected by the elder's gender. [2.3, 7.5]

<230> Ortega, S. T., Crutchfield, R. D., & Rushing, W. A. (1983). Race differences in elderly personal well-being: Friendship, family, and church. *Research on Aging, 5*, 101-118.

Data from a survey of 4,522 reveal that elderly blacks feel significantly greater personal well-being than whites. It appears that the association between race and life satisfaction is due, at least in part, to greater contact with church-related friends among black elderly. Race itself had little consequence. The black church may serve as the hub of a moral community, as a community of faith, or as a pseudo-extended family, all of which may foster a sense of well-being. [2.3, 5.1, 7.5]

<231> Page, R. M., & Cole G. E. (1991). Demographic predictors of self-reported loneliness in adults. *Psychological Reports, 68*, 939-945.

Examines the relative strengths of a series of demographic variables (gender, age, marital status, household income, educational attainment, race or ethnicity, employment status, and occupation) in explaining loneliness in a random sample of 8,634 adults. Logistic regression determined age as a predictor approaches significance, and gender is significant. Men report less loneliness. [2.3]

<232> Palinkas, L. A., Wingard, D. L., & Barrett-Connor, E. (1990). The biocultural context of social networks and depression among the elderly. *Social Science and Medicine, 30,* 441-447.

From a survey of 1,615 elderly persons age 65 and older, Beck Depression Inventory mean scores and rates of depressive symptoms are inversely associated with social networks and participation in voluntary associations and religious institutions. Depressive symptoms are inversely associated with the size of social networks. [2.3, 7.1, 7.5]

<233> Penning, M. J., & Strain, L. A. (1994). Gender differences in disability, assistance, and subjective well-being in later life. *Journal of Gerontology: Social Sciences, 49,* S202-S208.

Little work examines how much older men and women differ in functional disability and what ways they seek to deal with it. In data on 1,406 community dwelling elders in Manitoba, older men report less functional disability than women, and they report they receive less, if any assistance from others. For men with disability, the combination of disability and reliance on others or devices is associated with lowered feelings of well-being. Findings suggest that part of the reason for lowered feelings of well-being is the feeling of dependency (on others, on devices, on both). [2.1, 2.3]

<234> Phifer, J. F. (1990). Psychological distress and somatic symptoms after natural disaster: Differential vulnerability among older adults. *Psychology and Aging, 5,* 412-420.

In a panel study of 200 older adults, examines whether older adult flood victims are differentially vulnerable to increases in psychological and physical symptoms. Flood exposure increases in depressive, anxiety, and somatic symptoms 18 months post-flood. Within this older sample, men are at significantly greater risk for increases in psychological symptoms than women. This stands in contrast to prior work, which does not control for the initially higher rates of symptomalogy among women. Men may be more affected by financial difficulties, or women's social support may have helped them more fully recover than men 18 months post-flood. [2.3, 7.5]

<235> Powers, C. B., Wisocki, P. A., & Whitbourne, S. K. (1992). Age differences and correlates of worrying in young and elderly adults. *The Gerontologist, 32,* 82-88.

Consistent with prediction, a cross-sectional investigation shows elderly adults (N = 89) express significantly fewer worries than the college students (N = 74) about finances and social events. Both groups are equally worried about health issues. The elderly score higher on affect, in the external direction on locus of control, and more oriented toward the past and present than the future. Worry in the elderly is related to less favorable attitudes toward the future. For both age groups, an external locus of control is associated with higher worry scores. [2.3]

<236> Pruchno, R. A. (1990). The effects of help patterns on the mental health of spouse caregivers. *Research on Aging, 12,* 57-71.

Investigates the patterns of task assistance and social support received by 315 people who are the primary caregivers to spouses suffering from Alzheimer's Disease. Although spouse caregivers themselves are often old and frail, they continue to provide the bulk of care required by their impaired spouse--55% of the husbands, 60% of the wives are sole providers. Even when children are local, the overwhelming majority are not involved in providing assistance. Contrary to the hypothesis that back-up sources of support or confidants should buffer the primary caregiver from negative mental health effects, there is no relationship. [2.3, 7.5, 9.1]

<237> Quirouette, C., & Gold, D. P. (1992). Spousal characteristics as predictors of well-being in older couples. *International Journal of Aging and Human Development, 34,* 257-269.

Prior research demonstrates married men and women tend to have better mental health than unmarrieds, and the association between mental health and marriage is more salient for men. Theorizes the core marital roles (caregiving v. financial providing) promote more emotional responsiveness to a spouse's welfare in women than in men, and men's happiness rests on women's shoulders. Examines if spousal characteristics are less important determinants of psychological well-being for husbands (N = 60). Husbands' perceptions of the marriage and well-being significantly affect older wives' well-being, whereas wives' characteristics do not predict husbands' well-being. The results support the idea that differential emotional responsiveness of older husbands and help explain older men's better mental health. [2.3, 8.4]

<238> Russell, D. W., & Cutrona, C. E. (1991). Social support, stress, and depressive symptoms among the elderly: Test of a process model. *Psychology and Aging, 6,* 190-201.

Effects of social support, negative life events, and daily hassles on depressive symptoms are assessed in 301 adults age 65 and over, in person three times at 6-month intervals and by mail every month over a year period. Initial support predicts severity of depressive symptoms 12 months later. Support also predicts daily hassles but not number of major life events. Even though gender is often correlated with each construct studied, results do not differ for men and women. [2.3, 7.5]

<239> Ryff, C. D. (1989). In the eye of the beholder: Views of psychological well-being among middle-aged and older adults. *Psychology and Aging, 4,* 195-210.

Few studies investigate how adults define positive functioning. Interviews with a community sample of 171 middle-aged and older men and women provide data to examine views of the aging process and conceptions of well-being. Both age groups and sexes emphasize an "others orientation" (being a caring, compassionate person, and having good relationships) in defining well-being. When asked about life experiences, men answer more in terms of work experiences (promotions, career disappointments) or in terms of non-significant events, rather than family, death, relocation, and health. Men also differ from women on perceptions of change, reporting they have become more relaxed and mellowed, as opposed to more confident and assertive. These reports demonstrate an awareness of role changes, physical changes, and personal changes and a prominent sense of stability. [2.3, 2.4]

<240> Schulz, R., & Williamson, G. M. (1991). A 2-year longitudinal study of depression among Alzheimer's caregivers. *Psychology and Aging, 6*, 569-578.

A two-year (4 wave) longitudinal study shows strong evidence for patient decline and high levels of depressive symptomalogy among caregivers. Female caregivers report high, stable rates of depressive symptomalogy throughout the study, whereas male caregivers (who are most often older husbands) exhibited significant increases in depression over time. Also finds a decline in social support results in increased depression. [2.3, 9.1]

<241> Seccombe, K. (1987). Children: Their impact on the elderly in declining health. *Research on Aging, 9*, 312-326.

The effects of having children on the general happiness of elderly adults are identified from data on the 3,516 elders from the Retirement History Survey. Finds children do not contribute to the happiness of these adults nor lessen the impact of deteriorating health on well-being. This is true for both elderly men and women, despite the presumed differential importance of children in men's and women's lives. [2.3, 8.2]

<242> Siegel, J. M., & Kuykendall, D. H. (1990). Loss, widowhood, and psychological distress among the elderly. *Journal of Consulting and Clinical Psychology, 58*, 519-524.

Examines the psychological responses to recent nonspousal familial loss in a sample of 880 married or widowed adults age 65 or older. Finds nonspousal familial loss is associated with elevated levels of depressive symptomatology among men, but not women. Widowed men who report a loss within the past 6 months of a close family member are more depressed than their married counterparts. Widowers who experience a loss and do not belong to a church/temple are most depressed of all; all of these bereaved widowers score above the CES-D cutpoint for depression established in community studies. The importance of social ties in buffering distress and gender differences in coping with stress explain the findings. [2.3, 8.4]

<243> Silverstein, M., & Bengtson, V. L. (1991). Do close parent-child relations reduce the mortality risk of older parents? *Journal of Health and Social Behavior, 32*, 382-395.

Hypothesizes that close intergenerational relations have the capacity to reduce pathogenic stress among the elder parents, enchancing their ability to survive. Tests the direct and buffering effects of affectional solidarity over a 14-year period among 439 elderly parents. Hazard models indicate that greater intergenerational affect neither increases survival time nor buffers the experience of social decline. But the quality of relations does starve off mortality associated with social loss. Parents who feel close to their adult children are protected from the harmful stress of a social loss. [2.3, 7.5, 8.2]

<244> Simonsick, E. M. (1993). Relationship between husbands' health status and the mental health of older women. *Journal of Aging and Health*, 5, 319-337.

Investigates the codependency between husband's health and the mental health of wives age 65-75. Finds husband's health strongly predicts wives' mental health, and the negative effect is more pronounced when the wife already has poor or declining health. The effect of husband's health is a function of how his health affects marital quality and shared pursuits. Reductions in marital quality--level of interaction and consensus--undermine well-being more than burdens of caregiving. [2.3, 8.4]

<245> Sinnott, J. D. (1984-85). Stress, health, and mental health symptoms of older women and men. *International Journal of Aging and Human Development*, 20, 123-132.

Examines if a functioning, community-dwelling older adult appears symptomatic on mental health symptomalogy scales, and determines the relationship between symptoms, life-event stress, and physical health. Uses a sample of 364 elders age 60-90 who are associated with a senior center. Finds community-dwelling elders report relatively few symptoms, and men describe fewer. Men with incongruity between actual and expected masculinity on the Bem Sex Role Inventory are role-conflicted, but their gender role conflict is not related to symptoms or stress. Only for men is age related to life event stress and mental health symptoms; older men experience more stress than the less elderly, but fewer mental health symptoms. Sicker men experience more stress than healthier men, but stress is unrelated to symptoms. [1.3, 2.3]

<246> Smallegan, M. (1989). Level of depressive symptoms and life stresses for culturally diverse older adults. *The Gerontologist*, 29, 45-50.

Studies often find men have less depression than women, but some research finds the opposite. Research on whether or not depressive episodes are precipitated by life events also has not provided unequivocal findings. Conduces interviews with 181 people age 65 and older to determine the relation between depressive symptoms and life stresses. Somewhat more women than men have more depressive symptoms, however there is no reliable gender difference. When living with a spouse and disability level are controlled, even the trend that women are more depressed disappears. Life events--particularly moving, marital change, and arguments with family and friends--are related to level of depression before and after controlling for physical disability and living with a spouse. [2.3]

<247> Solomon, K. (1982). The older man. In K. Solomon & N. B. Levy (Eds.), *Men in transition: Theory and therapy* (pp. 205-240). New York: Plenum.

Reviews the special characteristics, problems, and needs of older men. The issues range from the direct effects on life expectancy to psychosocial factors that influence the welfare of the older man in American society. Stress and coping among older men is the major focus of the chapter, and the author uses a continuity perspective to explain the stability of gender and gender roles across the life span. [2.2, 2.3]

<248> Solomon, K. (1981). Masculine gender role and its implications for the life expectancy of older men. *Journal of the American Geriatrics Society,* **29,** 297-301.

Theorizes that older men face stressors that the masculine role has not prepared them for (e.g., retirement, widowhood, and diseases and disability), and men can manifest the stress in the use of drugs, alcohol, cigarettes, and caffeine. Examines how six dimensions of traditional masculinity may be related to stress-related disorders more prevalent among older men. These masculinity norms affect the responses of men to stress and play a role in limiting the lifespan. Should older men's gender role change toward androgyny, one could expect men to live as long as women do. [1.4, 2.3]

<249> Spiro, A. 3rd., Schnurr, P. P., & Aldwin, C. M. (1994). Combat-related posttraumatic stress disorder symptoms in older men. *Psychology and Aging,* **9,** 17-26.

Close to 25 percent of men age 55 and older have served in combat. Investigates the relationship of combat exposure to post traumatic stress disorder symptoms among 1,120 veterans who are participants in the Normative Aging Study. Over half of the World War II and one-of-every-five Korean conflict veterans report combat exposure, and post traumatic stress disorder symptoms are strongest in the World War II veteran cohort. Exposed to moderate or heavy combat adds 13 times greater risk of symptoms. Concludes that military service in general, and combat exposure in particular, are "hidden" risk factors in the study of aging men. [2.3, 12.2]

<250> Stull, D. E. (1988). A dyadic approach to predicting well-being in later life. *Research on Aging,* **10,** 81-101.

Determines the importance of a number of variables previously found to predict well-being (e.g., income, health, social interaction) for happiness at pre- and post-retirement for husbands and wives. Finds husbands and wives do have different predictors of happiness. For husbands, health, household income, and wife's happiness are predictors, and interaction with family is not. Contrary to expectations, neither interaction with family nor husband's health predict wives' happiness. Concludes that including the wife's characteristics is central to understanding husbands' well-being. [2.3, 8.4]

<251> Szinovacz, M. (1992). Is housework good for retirees? *Family Relations,* **41,** 230-238.

Examines when postretirement household involvement contributes to or decreases husbands' and wives' retirement adjustment. Notable gender differences are observed. For women (N = 275), high postretirement housework covaries with positive adjustment to the retirement transition, but the causal direction is ambiguous. Men (N = 336) continue to view their participation in household work as a "helping role," and the relationship between housework and adaptation is contingent on such factors as involvement is an expression of love, spouse's health, and marital relationship reasons. Men's housework also enhances retirement adjustment when their health prevents them from other activities. [1.4, 2.3, 8.4, 10.2]

<252> Tesch, S. A., Whitbourne, S. K., & Nehrke, M. F. (1981). Friendship, social interaction and subjective well-being of older men in an institutional setting. *International Journal of Aging and Human Development, 13*, 317-327.

Investigates the effect of informal social interaction on subjective well-being for 54 men residing in a nursing home. Finds the hypothesized positive correlation between morale and frequency of social interaction with persons outside the residential facility, but men's friendships within the institution are not related to morale. As expected, older men who report an overall change in frequency of social interaction show lower well-being. Results conform to a continuity model of aging, where maintenance of social interaction is related to subjective well-being. [2.3, 7.3, 7.5, 11.1]

<253> Thomas, L. E., & Chambers, K. O. (1989). Phenomenology of life satisfaction among elderly men: Quantitative and qualitative views. *Psychology and Aging, 4*, 284-289.

Compares standardized measures of subjective well-being with qualitative analysis of life satisfaction for 100 elderly men for New Delhi and London. When the standardized, structured measures of well-being are use, one concludes that the English and Indian elderly in this sample differ very little. One might conclude that the common experiences of aging are more important than major cultural differences. However, from the open-ended interviews, it is clear that the English and Indian men live in different psychological and social worlds. Not only do they differ in the overarching themes, but they differ in several of the dimensions often mentioned as constituting life satisfaction, particularly convergence between desired and achieved goals. [2.3]

<254> Thompson, L. W., Gallagher-Thompson, D., Futterman, A., Gilewski, M. J., & Peterson, J. (1991). The effects of late-life spousal bereavement over a 30-month interval. *Psychology & Aging, 6*, 434-441.

Grief, depression, and general psychopathology are studied in widows and widowers over a two-and-one-half-year period following death of the spouse. Severity of depression and psychopathology reported at 2 months post-loss diminishes to nonsignificant levels at 12 and 30 months. Men report less distress (depression and psychopathology) but not for grief at 2 and 12 months. Results indicate that grief persists for at least 30 months in older men and women who have lost their spouse. [2.3]

<255> Tran, T. V., Wright, R. Jr., & Chatters, L. (1991). Health, stress, psychological resources, and subjective well-being among older blacks. *Psychology and Aging, 6*, 100-108.

Examines the relationships among sociodemographic characteristics, health status, stress, psychological resources, and subjective well-being (SWB) among the black elderly. Evaluates a structural equation model of SWB with data from the 1979-1980 National Survey of Black Americans. Finds SWB is multidetermined, directly effected by personal efficacy, self-esteem, poor health status, stressful life events, being married and older. Gender and living conditions, measured by income and education, do not directly determine black elders sense of well-being, but they have indirect effects through intermediate factors (e.g., martial and health status). [2.3]

<256> Umberson, D., Wortman, C. B., & Kessler, R. C. (1992). Widowhood and depression: Explaining long-term gender differences in vulnerability. *Journal of Health and Social Behavior, 33*, 10-24.

Investigates how widowhood contributes to enduring depression and why men and women experience widowhood differently. Interviews with 3,614 persons--787 widowed, reveal that the men are widowed for a shorter period of time than women, and the effects of widowhood appears to lessen over time. Gender differences in primary sources of strain are closely linked to prior gender differences in marital roles; thus, for example, men are less likely to experience vulnerability as a result of financial strain. What appears to be a gender difference in vulnerability to the same life event turns out to occur because widowhood affects men and women differently. [2.3]

<257> Vaillant, G. E. (1994). "Successful aging" and psychological well-being: Evidence from a 45-year study. In E. Thompson (Ed.), *Older men's lives* (pp. 22-41). Thousand Oaks, CA: Sage Publications.

Examines longitudinally two general outcomes of "successful aging" -- physical health and psychosocial health -- for the 173 survivors of the Grant Study of Harvard under-graduates in the 1940s. Finds 22 percent of the men continue to report excellent health to age 63; many others live with chronic illness and many experience minor problems such as hypertension. By age 65, only 37 of the men report no negative outcomes in three domains of psychosocial health. Concludes that "successful aging" (remaining in good physical and psychological health) is related to sibling closeness, career success, and avoidance of alcohol abuse. But there are many discontinuities, and what predicts healthy men at age 65 is largely undetermined. [1.5, 2.2, 2.3]

<258> Wheaton, B. (1990). Life transitions, role histories, and mental health. *American Sociological Review, 55*, 209-223.

Develops a model which envisions life transition events as nonproblematic, even beneficial to mental health, when preceded by chronic role problems--a case where more stress is actually relief from existing stress. Nine transition events are studied (e.g., first marriage, job promotion, having a child, job loss, divorce, retirement, widowhood). Results support the hypothesized "cathartic effect," where men entering retirement from high stress work contexts experience fewer symptoms. Men leaving low work stress situations report an modest increase in symptoms. Concludes that retirement is less of a problem and more a relief for many. All three late life transitions (retirement, death of a spouse, child moving out) reveal a stress-relief effect. [2.3,10.2]

<259> Zisook, S., Shuchter, S. R., Sledge, P., & Mulvihill, M. (1993). Aging and bereavement. *Journal of Geriatric Psychiatry and Neurology, 6*, 137-143.

Compares the severity and types of grief responses of widows and widowers of different ages over the first year of bereavement. Results strongly suggest that older widows and widowers perceive themselves as adjusting better to their loss (less depression and fewer anxiety symptoms) than younger counterparts. Older widowers are not any more disadvantaged, as would be predicted by certain stereotypes and "clinical wisdoms." [2.3]

SELF-PERCEPTIONS OF HEALTH

<260> Arber, S., & Ginn, J. (1993). Gender and inequalities in health in later life. *Social Science & Medicine, 36,* 33-46.

Argues that research on inequalities in health has largely neglected elders--the age-group with the greatest ill-health. Analyzes data from the British General Household Survey for variation in health of elderly men and women by class and material circumstances. Finds elderly men assess their own health more positively than women, and men are much less disadvantaged in functional disability. Also finds inequalities in health are equally pronounced for men and women in later life. Elders who live in advantaged material circumstances, in terms of income and housing tenure, report significantly better health (self-assessed and functional disability), after controlling for age and class. [2.4, 12.2]

<261> Ferraro, K. F. (1993). Are black older adults health-pessimistic? *Journal of Health and Social Behavior, 34,* 201-214.

Investigates if the more extensive health problems of older blacks lead to a pessimistic outlook on health. Data from the 1984 Health Interview Survey (N= 3,237) demonstrate that older blacks report more functional morbidity than whites, more negative health assessments, and are less likely to engage in health promotion. Black men did not report as many health problems as expected, suggesting that those who survive to enter their sixties are in robust health, and their life expectancy eventually exceeds that of white men. They appear to engage in more efforts to promote and preserve their health, and they are not health-pessimistic, but black women are. [2.1, 2.4]

<262> Gibson, R. C. (1991). Race and self-reported health of elderly persons. *Journals of Gerontology: Social Sciences, 46,* S235-S242.

Analyzes the comparability of black and white elders' self-evaluations of health by evaluating differences in the structure and measurement of six self-reports of health. Data are on 529 blacks and 557 whites age 55-96 from the Americans' Changing Lives study. The cognitive illness-reporting process, overall, may be the same for blacks and whites. Culture and race affect the illness-reporting process in specific stages rather than as a whole. Subjective interpretation is a less valid measure of actual health state for blacks, perhaps because self-defined health is more multidetermined. [2.4]

<263> Hansell, S., & Mechanic, D. (1991). Body awareness and self-assessed health among older adults. *Journal of Aging and Health, 3,* 473-492.

Finds in a longitudinal study of 1,124 older adult members of a health maintenance organization that higher levels of body awareness parallel decreases in self-assessed health over time, after controlling for physical and psychological health status, gender, age, and education. Men have greater longitudinal increases in body awareness (attention to body sensations and symptoms) than women, perhaps because they have more frequent reminders of their own mortality through their own illness and through losses within their personal networks. Body awareness affects propensity to recognize health problems. [2.4, 2.5]

<264> Hardy, M. A., & Pavalko, E. K. (1986). Internal structure of self-reported health measures among older male workers and retirees. *Journal of Health and Social Behavior, 27,* 346-357.

Examines the structure of the self-reported health measures in the National Longitudinal Surveys of Older Men. Data obtained on 1,551 employed or formerly employed white men age 55 to 69 in four white-collar and four blue-collar occupational categories reveal that there is no difference between white-and blue-collar workers in the frequency of work-limiting health condition. Concludes that characteristics of the person, as opposed to characteristics of the workplace, predict a work-limiting health condition more accurately. It is also noted that self-reported health status reflects the evaluative context within which the worker responds to interview questions. [2.4]

<265> Hooker, K. (1992). Possible selves and perceived health in older adults and college students. *Journals of Gerontology: Psychological Sciences, 47,* P85-P95.

Predicts that health-related selves would be predominant among older adults, but not college students, and that self-regulatory aspects of possible selves would be related to perceived health. As predicted, older adults are more likely to have possible selves in the realm of health. Regression analyses indicate that outcome expectancy for a hoped-for self is positively related to perceived health, whereas amount of time spent thinking about a hoped-for possible self is negatively related to perceived health. These relationships are no longer significant for a feared possible self, indicating likely differences in the way elders' self-regulatory processes operate in service of positive v. negative goals for self. [1.1, 2.4]

<266> Krause, N. (1987). Satisfaction with social support and self-rated health in older adults. *The Gerontologist, 27,* 301-308.

Determines whether elders satisfied with the amount of different types of social support received are more likely to rate their health as better than elders dissatisfied with the support they receive. Data from 325 older adults reveal satisfaction with support (both tangible or emotional, but not informational) is an important determinant of self-perceived health and depressed affect. Men report receiving a good deal less tangible and emotional support than women, nonetheless the relationship between satisfaction with the support received and subjective health remains significant after controlling for gender and the amount of support. [2.3, 2.4, 7.5]

<267> Nuttbrock, L. (1986). Socialization to the chronic sick role in later life. *Research on Aging, 8,* 368-387.

Examines sick role retention among older adults. Using an interactionist framework and studying physically impaired older people age 55-85, sick role socialization is found mirroring the role casting of others and in portraying sickness in pursuit of social support or relief from strain. Role casting is caused by the elder's incapacity, not age or gender as hypothesized by labeling theory. Nor did casting cause the elder to adopt an identity as sick. Sick role retention is more common among older men, in part because they are treated as sick by others, and because of their own health status. [2.4, 2.5]

<268> Rakowski, W., Mor, V., & Hiris, J. (1991). **The association of self-rated health with two-year mortality in a sample of well elderly.** *Journal of Aging and Health, 3,* 527-545.

Investigates longitudinally self-assessed health as a predictor of mortality among 1,252 men and women age 70 and older. Logistic regression shows independent predictive effects with higher mortality for age (older), gender (men), and having no children or siblings. Self-assessments of health also should be taken seriously, especially if comments are made over successive appointments or across questions addressing quality of life. [2.1, 2.4]

<269> Rodin, J., & McAvay, G. (1992). **Determinants of change in perceived health in a longitudinal study of older adults.** *Journals of Gerontology: Psychological Sciences, 47,* P373-P384.

Determines predictors of a decline in perceived health in a longitudinal study of 251 men and women age 62 and older. Analyses reveal new illness, greater physician visits, and worsening preexisting conditions are associated with declines in perceived health, after controlling for baseline illnesses and medication use. Lower life satisfaction and greater depression also are predictive. Although no differences in men's and women's overall depression are observed, depression influences the sense of self more in men. Prior level of depression and an increase in depression predict a negative change in perceived health for men. [2.4]

<270> Ross, C. E., & Bird, C. E. (1994). **Sex stratification and health lifestyle: Consequences for men's and women's perceived health.** *Journal of Health and Social Behavior, 35,* 161-178.

Investigates what explains the pattern of men reporting better health than women until later life, when the gap closes. Using data from 2,031 adults age 18-90, a gender difference in the components of class--labor and lifestyles--explains the effect of gender on health across the life course and men's acquired health advantage. Men are less likely to be involved in unpaid domestic labor. The are more likely to work for pay, work full-time, have greater subjective work rewards, greater incomes, and less economic hardship or levels of distress. They exercise more. After age 54, however, men's health advantage diminishes and women's appears. [2.4]

<271> Roy, P. G., & Storand, M. (1989). **Older adults' perceptions of psychopathology.** *Psychology and Aging, 4,* 369-371.

Tests the hypothesis that women would rate symptoms of psychopathology as more severe than men because of their greater sensitivity to such pathology. Forty older women and 40 men age 60-78 read fictional case descriptions of a health person and of five individuals with paranoia, depression, dementia, hypocondriasis, and alcohol abuse. Half read descriptions of an older man. The hypothesis that older men would rate the psychopathology less severely is not supported. The findings suggest that older women are no more likely to perceive psychopathology than are older men. [2.4]

<272> Stoller, E. P. (1993). Interpretations of symptoms by older people: A health diary study of illness behavior. *Journal of Aging and Health, 5*, 58-81.

Examines interpretations of symptoms experienced in a probability sample of 667 community-based older men and women living in upstate New York. Few respondents believe their symptoms are definitely serious, yet the majority experience some uncertainty regarding the potential seriousness of at least one symptom. People who rate their health as poor report more negative interpretations of specific symptoms and are less likely to dismiss symptoms. Stressful life events have minimal effect on symptom interpretation, whereas social support has an indirect effect -- people with support are less likely to interpret symptoms as serious. Contrary to prediction, occupying multiple roles is positively related to assessments of symptom pain and interference. [2.4]

<273> Thompson, L. W., Brekenridge, J. N., Gallagher, D., & Peterson, J. (1984). Effects of bereavement on self-perceptions of physical health in elderly widows and widowers. *Journal of Gerontology, 39*, 309-314.

Much is known about how stressful life events affect physical well-being, but the extent to which elders are likely to suffer deteriorating health as a consequence of the loss of a spouse is uncertain.   Describes self-perceptions of physical health status for 99 bereaved men and 113 women two months after their spouse's death.   Recently bereaved elderly adults are more likely than other elders to report new illnesses, the beginning of new medication, or increasing dosage. Contrary to expectation, bereaved elder men do not report greater morbidity than women, yet this finding may be an artifact of the temporal proximity between spousal loss and assessment of health. [2.4]

<274> Uhlmann, R. F., Pearlman, R. A., & Cain, K. C. (1988). Physicians' and spouses' predictions of elderly patients' resuscitation preferences. *Journal of Gerontology: Medical Sciences, 43*, M115-M121.

Studies the accuracy of 105 primary care physicians and 90 spouses in predicting 258 elderly outpatients' preferences for cardiopulmonary resuscitation. Accuracy of substituted judgment, in which surrogate decision makers approximate patients' wishes, does not exceed that predicted by chance, even though three-quarters of physicians and spouses believed their predictions are accurate. Physicians underestimate and spouses overestimate decisions. [2.4, 12.2]

<275> Wolinsky, F. D., & Johnson, R. J. (1992). Perceived health status and mortality among older men and women. *Journals of Gerontology: Social Sciences, 47*, S304-S312.

The possible effect of perceived health on mortality has many post hoc explanations. Examines the relationship of health status and mortality for the 1,599 men and 2,904 women using data from the Longitudinal Study on Aging. Based on hierarchical logistic regressions which first introduces demographic, socioeconomic, health status, and psychosocial factors, finds the direct effect of health is still present. Men in poor health are significantly more likely to die than those in excellent health, all other things being equal. For women, subjective reports of fair and poor health predict death. [2.1, 2.4]

HEALTH BEHAVIOR

<276> Blumenthal, J. A., Emery, C. F., Madden, D. J., George, L. K., Coleman, R. E., Riddle, M. W., McKee, D. C., Reasoner, J., & Williams, R. S. (1989). Cardiovascular and behavioral effects of aerobic exercise training in healthy older men and women. *Journals of Gerontology: Medical Sciences, 44,* **M147-M157.**

Examines the cardiovascular and behavioral adaptations associated with a 4-month program of aerobic exercise training in older men and women. Notes that physical exercise has become increasingly popular as a method of health enhancement, however the paucity of information on older persons raises concern about the potential hazards of unsupervised exercise. Demonstrates that 4 months of exercise produced 12 percent improvement in peak oxygen consumption and 13 percent in anaerobic threshold. Other favorable changes included lower diastolic blood pressure levels. Few psychological changes could be attributed to exercise training. [2.5]

<277> Catania, J. A., Turner, H., Kegeles, S. M., Stall, R., Pollack, L., & Coates, T. (1989). Older Americans and AIDS: Transmission risks and primary prevention research needs. *The Gerontologist, 29,* **373-381.**

Calls attention to the growing number of AIDS cases among older Americans age 50 and older. If monogamy was the norm among older individuals, the AIDS epidemic for this population may be limited. However, finds recent cohorts of older heterosexual men exhibit a higher prevalence of extramarital sexual activity than older men of the past. Also finds a sizable minority of older gays are not lifetime monogamous, and because most older homosexual men continue to be sexually active, their risks also increase with sexual activity. [2.5, 3.2]

<278> Connell, C. M., Fisher, E. B., & Houston, C. A. (1992). Relationships among social support, diabetes outcomes, and morale for older men and women. *Journal of Aging and Health, 4,* **77-100.**

Gauges whether diabetes-specific social support is better related to diabetes outcomes than general social support, and whether self-care behavior influences morale. Data are from 81 community-dwelling men and 110 women age 60 and older with non-insulin-dependent diabetes. For men, not women, support specific to one's regiment affects metabolic control by increasing self-care behavior. Married men who perceive high levels of available support from family and friends report high morale, as did men who are in better metabolic control. Concludes that types of support and psychosocial endpoints may be more important markers for older men than physiological indicator of diabetes control. [2.1, 2.5, 7.5]

<279> Davis, R. M., Rosenberg, A. M., Connell, C. M., & Fisher, E. B. Jr. (1993). Interest in cardiovascular health promotion programs among corporate retirees. *Behavior, Health, and Aging, 3,* **87-99.**

Employers and insurers are increasingly interested in promoting good health among retirees as health care costs rise. In a sample of 756 retirees age 55 and older, 71 percent express interest in health promotion activities, and consistent with prior research, younger age, higher education, and retiring later are better predictors of health promotion involvement than self-report health. These findings underscore how sociodemographic and cohort characteristics influence health promotion activities more than health behavior being a rational response to health status. [2.1, 2.5, 10.2, 12.2]

<280> Dodge, J. A., Clark, N. M., Janz, N. K., Liang, J., & Schork, M. A. (1993). Nonparticipation of older adults in a heart disease self-management project. *Research on Aging, 15,* 220-237.

Tries to clarify what factors influence elders to take part in service and education programs and participate in studies which evaluate them. The hypothesis is that those who agree to participate in the evaluation of a heart disease self-management program are representative of the larger population of older cardiac patients. Finds, however, participants are most likely men, with more formal education, more worried about their heart condition, and less likely to perceive the help that is available. [2.5, 12.2]

<281> Duffy, M. D., & MacDonald, E. (1990). Determinants of functional health of older persons. *The Gerontologist, 30,* 503-509.

Investigates the relationships among self esteem, health locus of control, health promotion behavior, perceived health, and functional health ratings in 179 men and women age 65-99. Discovers exercise and nutrition are more critical health promotion activities for elders than some prior research has suggested. For the three groups of unmarried men (the widowed, divorced, and never-married), more exercise, better health status, higher self esteem, and an internal health locus of control are all interdependent. Older men who are healthy and physically active are more prevalent among the men without a spouse. [1.3, 2.5]

<282> Emery, C. F., Hauch, E. R., & Blumenthal, J. A. (1992). Exercise adherence or maintenance among older adults: 1-Year follow-up study. *Psychology and Aging, 7,* 466-470.

Reviews and discusesses studies of elders' poor exercise adherence in structured programs as well as exercise maintenance outside the program. A follow-up evaluation of 85 of 101 older men and women who participate in an earlier randomized study of aerobic exercise finds almost all (94%) report that they continued with physical activity. Gender did not predict exercise behavior or variance in energy expenditure. [2.5]

<283> Hawley, P. J., & Klauber, M. R. (1988). Health practices and perceptions of social support in persons over age sixty. *Journal of Applied Gerontology, 7,* 205-230.

Investigates the health practices and perceptions of social support for 23 men and 41 women age 60-75 who were either inactive, moderately active, or active. Elders who are satisfied with their interpersonal relationships engaged in more healthful practices than those who are not satisfied. Health practices have a stronger relation to satisfaction with social support received than with the number of people in a support network. The strongest link to health behavior is communication with other people. Men show significantly higher correlations between health habits and satisfaction with social support through sharing than women. [2.5, 7.5]

<284> Hickey, T., Rakowski, W., & Julius, M. (1988). Preventive health practices among older men and women. *Research on Aging*, 10, 315-328.

Examines the preventive health practices of older men and women using interviews with a community sample of 172 elders age 64-96. Although men and women differ in the patterns of illness, gender differences are found on just 10 of 37 health practices. Findings are interpreted as men become more preventive with age; the age-related mortality risks faced by men may influence health behavior in late life. As likely, men may be less gender role stereotypic in later life, and health care decisions and health maintenance behaviors may be less determined by gender characteristics. [2.5]

<285> Kamen-Siegel, L., Rodin, J., Seligman, M., & Dwyer, J. W. (1991). Explanatory style and cell-mediated immunity in elderly men and women. *Health Psychology, 10*, 229-235.

Investigates the relationship between a pessimistic explanatory style--the belief that negative events are caused by internal, stable, and global factors--and immunocompetence in 26 older adults age 62-82. Two measures of cell-mediated immunity (T-helper cell/T-suppressor cell ratio and T-lymphocyte response to mitogen challenge) are lower in individuals with a pessimistic style, controlling for the influence of current health, depression, medication, recent weight change, sleep, and alcohol use. A relative increase in the percentage of T-suppressor cells appears to underlie this immunosuppression. A pessimistic style might be an important risk factor among older people in the early course of certain immune-mediated diseases. [2.5]

<286> Koenig, H. G. (1991). Religion and prevention of illness in later life. *Prevention in Human Services*, 10, 69-89.

Reviews available research investigating the relationship between religion and health in later life. Presents the equation that traditional Judeo-Christian beliefs and behaviors are likely to be positively related to adjustment and well-being in late life. Discusses the implications of religion as a coping strategy and the mediating effects of mental health on physical health outcomes and health care use. [2.3, 2.5, 5.1]

<287> Krause, N., Goldenhar, L., Liang, J., Jay, G., & Maeda, D. (1993). Stress and exercise among the Japanese elderly. *Social Science and Medicine, 36*, 1429-1441.

The recurring finding that stressful life events depress daily mood and erode feelings of well-being in later life is almost exclusively based on Western cultures. Tries to replicate and examines the relationships among stress, social support, physical exercise, and depressive symptoms with data from a nationwide sample of older adults in Japan. Finds social support promotes more frequent exercise, more frequent physical exercise is associated with less distress, and men report fewer symptoms of depressed affect. However, gender is unrelated to exercise habits. [2.3, 2.5]

<288> Leigh, J. P., & Fries, J. F. (1992-93). **Associations among healthy habits, age, gender, and education in a sample of retirees.** *International Journal of Aging And Human Development, 36,* **139-155**.

Theorizes that morbidity and mortality may be as tied to individuals' health behaviors as their access to medical care. Investigates the relationships among elders' healthy habits, age, gender, and education using data from a sample of 1,864 Bank of America employees in 1987. Important gender differences are found. Men are more like to drink and less likely to use seat belts, or eat foods high in fiber, yet they are more likely than women to exercise and less likely to smoke. [2.5]

<289> Luptak, M. K., & Boult, C. (1994). **A method for increasing elders' use of advance directives.** *The Gerontologist, 34,* **409-412**.

Studies the effectiveness of an interdisciplinary intervention designed to help ambulatory frail elders (average age 75) to record an advance directive, which states how medical decisions should be made if the patient should become mentally or physically unable to choose options. Finds the intervention encouraged 24 (70 percent) of the 34 elders to record a directive, yet men are significantly less likely to record an advance directive. [2.5, 12.2]

<290> McAuley, E., Courneya, K. S., & Lettunich, J. (1991). **Effects of acute and long-term exercise on self-efficacy responses in sedentary, middle-aged males and females.** *The Gerontologist, 31,* **534-542**.

Exercise is often suggested to be the single health practice most strongly associated with health and longevity among the age. From a psychological perspective, the effects of regular exercise on the individual's sense of perceived control and well-being are important. Examines the effects of exercise on perceptions of personal efficacy in 81 sedentary, middle-aged males and females (age 45-64). Finds significant increases in efficacy performance and beliefs following exercise (bicycle ergometry). Men have initially greater self-perceptions of their physical capabilities than women prior to the exercise program, yet women make dramatic increases in efficacy during the exercise program, equaling or surpassing those of men. Concludes that preconceptions of abilities seemed based on prior experiences and socialization, yet they accuracy is equivocal. [2.5]

<291> O'Brien S. J., & Conger P. R. (1991). **No time to look back: approaching the finish line of life's course.** *International Journal of Aging and Human Development, 33,* **75-87**.

Gerontologists label older men and women who do not follow the normal aging pattern of reduced physical activity and declining health as "successfully aging" adults. Hypothesizes that competitive and sport-involved elder persons represent a kind of elderly elite who may exhibit special psychological characteristics that explain their active approach to late life. Examines in a qualitative study the personal life philosophy among participants at seniors' games. Finds evidence that sport and physical recreation may be an important type of coping strategy for some elderly adults who find life meaning and a sense of achievement in challenging themselves physically. [2.5]

<292> Rakowski, W., Julius, M., Hickey, T., & Halter, J. B. (1987). Correlates of preventive health behavior in late life. *Research on Aging*, *9*, 331-355.

Interviews 172 community-dwelling elders age 64-96 to examine correlates of their preventive-oriented, health-related practices. Four health practice patterns are investigated -- information-seeking, regular health routines, medical and self-examinations, and risk avoidance. Results indicate older men have poorer health practices than women. [2.5]

<293> Rakowski, W., Julius, M., Hickey, T., Verbrugge, L. M., & Halter, J. B. (1988). Daily symptoms and behavioral responses: Results of a health diary with older adults. *Medical Care*, *26*, 278-297.

Studies symptom experiences, the accompanying pain and discomfort, and the actions taken in response to them over a two-week period using interview data and a self-kept diary for 60 community-dwelling men and 82 women age 62-94. Men take a less active response to symptoms than women, particularly in the area of personal care. Symptom-related actions and preventive health behaviors are not predictive of seeking professional assistance. [2.5]

<294> Stoller, E. P. (1993). Gender and the organization of lay health care: A socialist-feminist perspective. *Journal of Aging Studies*, *7*, 151-170.

Gender and the organization of lay health care are examined from a feminist perspective. A sample of 667 elders is interviewed as well as complete health diaries for 21 days. Among the married, 75 percent of the husbands indicate that their wives are their only lay consultants, compared to 42 percent of wives who rely exclusively on their husbands. Widowed men are less likely than widowed women to report lay referral networks, yet both are equally likely to select women consultants. Several theoretical approaches commonly used to explain the differentials between men's and women's unpaid care are systematically reviewed. [2.4, 2.5]

<295> Wallhagen, M. I., Strawbridge, W. J., Kaplan, G. A., & Cohen, R. D. (1944). Impact of internal health locus of control on health outcomes for older men and women: A longitudinal perspective. *The Gerontologist*, *34*, 299-306.

Investigates the relationship between baseline internal health locus of control and six-year change in physical functioning in 147 older men and 209 older women. Finds distinct gender differences. For men, the effect of locus of control on change in physical functioning depends on their level of functioning at baseline, and only affected men with lower baseline functioning. Internal health locus of control was not associated with most health behaviors, but may influence individual daily events that affect functioning over time. [2.3, 2.4, 2.5]

<296> Ward, S. E., Goldberg, N., Miller-McCauley, V., Mueller, C., Nolan, A., Pawlik-Plank, D., Robbins, A., Stormoen, D., & Weissman, D. E. (1993). Patient-related barriers to management of cancer pain. *Pain*, *52*, 319-324.

Patients' reluctance to report pain and to use analgesics are major barriers to pain management. This research examines beliefs that may be barriers to optimal pain management. Both men and women who are older, less educated, or have lower incomes are more likely to have reticence about reporting pain or taking medication. Men are less concerned about side effects than women. [2.5, 12.2]

<297> Woodward, N. J., & Wallston, B. S. (1987). Age and health care beliefs: Self-efficacy as a mediator of low desire for control. *Psychology and Aging, 2,* 3-8.

Age differences in health care beliefs are poorly documented. Examines the relationships between age and desire for control, information, and self-efficacy in a sample of 116 adults age 20 to 99. Individuals over 60 desire less health-related control than do young adults, and they prefer health professional make decisions for them. Desire for health-related information shows a similar pattern but is not reliable. The findings suggest that individuals more at risk for chronic illness and hospitalization are also least likely to take an active role in their health care. [2.5]

3

Sexuality

— ♦ —

SEXUAL HEALTH

<298> Barber, H. R. K., Lewis, M. I., Long, J., Whitehead, E. D., & Butler, R. N. (1989). Sexual problems in the elderly, II: Men's vs. women's. *Geriatrics*, *44*, 75-78.

Summarizes a panel discussion of the major sexual problems experienced by older men and women, and the role of the primary care physician in treating each dysfunction. Prevention of cardiovascular risk factors is one way of preventing vasculogenic impotence. Proposes that before an impotent patient is referred for psychotherapy, it is important that the physician have a thorough physical workup. Vascular surgery is successful only in about 50-60 percent of carefully selected patients. Sex counseling and sex therapy are very important; older men need to be aware that changes in sexual response are a normal part of aging. Primary care physicians may address such problems in one or two discussions with the family, or they may wish to refer the patient to a religious counselor or a family therapist. [3.1, 12..2]

<299> Blessing, J. D., & Warren, M. M. (1993). Effective treatment options for men with impotence. *Journal of the American Academy of Physician Assistants*, *6*, 267-274.

Reviews for physician assistants the fact that impotence, or erection dysfunction, is no longer accepted as a consequence of aging, disease, injury, or disability. Men are living longer, have healthier lifestyles, and do not automatically resign themselves to the loss of sexual activity. The physiologic aspects and dysfunctions of penile erection are better understood, and this enables clinicians to identify those men who will benefit from treatment. Patient education and inclusion of the sexual partner are defined as important for treatment success. [3.1, 12.2]

<300> Butler, R. N., Lewis, M. I., Hoffman, E., & Whitehead, E. D. (1994). Love and sex after 60: How physical changes affect intimate expression. *Geriatrics*, *49* (Sept), 20-27.

Discusses the dissonance arising from negative folklore about elders' sexuality and from their internalization of these cultural scripts, and encourages physicians to be aware of these special concerns from their patients. Sexuality is too often discussed only in terms of the physical aspects, and many sexual problems are not the result of normal changes related to aging, but rather the result of co-morbidities and medical side-effects. The urge for sexual gratification decreases with age for men, and the hardness and duration of the erection also diminish due to age-related physical changes, however this present and opportunity to move beyond "penis-in-vagina" centered sex. Yet, to be sexually active, some older people are thwarted by social or emotional obstacles to intimacy. Older men and physicians need to distinguish between performance v. intimacy and not always consider erectile dysfunction as ultimately important. [3.1, 12.2]

<301> Butler, R. N., Lewis, M. I., Hoffman, E., & Whitehead, E. D. (1994). Love and sex after 60: How to evaluate and treat the impotent older man. *Geriatrics, 49* (Oct), 27-32.

Discusses impotence, the sexual problem for which older men are most likely to seek help from their physicians. Complaints of impotence are likely signs of underlying morbidity such as diabetes or coronary artery disease, and physicians must determine if there is a primary and treatable cause for the impotence. Vascular problems are the most common cause, affecting 80 percent of older men who are impotent. The accepted 1994 treatment modality is the intracavernosal injection of pharmacologic agents into the penis by the patient, who is taught how by his physician. This has tended to replace penile implants. Physicians and patients, however, must recognize that performance anxiety compounds the dysfunction. [3.1, 12.2]

<302> Feldman, H. A., Goldstein, I., Hatzichristou, D. G., Krane, R. J., & McKinlay, J. B. (1994). Impotence and its medical and psychosocial correlates: Results of the Massachusetts Male Aging Study. *Journal of Urology, 151,* 54-61.

Normative data on the prevalence of impotence and physiological and psychosocial correlates in a general population are provided. Data are from the Massachusetts Male Aging Study. The combined prevalence of minimal, moderate and complete impotence is 52 percent. The prevalence of complete impotence triples from 5 to 15 percent between age 40 and 70 years. Age is the variable most strongly associated with impotence. After adjustment for age, a higher probability of impotence is directly correlated with heart disease, hypertension, diabetes, and indexes of anger and depression, and inversely correlated with serum dehydroepiandrosterone, high density lipoprotein cholesterol and an index of dominant personality. These findings underscore how impotence is a major health concern of the high prevalence, is strongly associated with age, has multiple determinants, including some risk factors for vascular disease, and may be due partly to modifiable para-aging phenomena. [2.1, 3.1, 6.2]

<303> Lewis, J. H. (1992). Treatment options for men with sexual dysfunction. *Journal of ET Nursing, 19,* 131-142.

Reviews the sexual dysfunction in older male patients ET nurses must be prepared to address. Erectile dysfunction can occur in men at any age, but it is more common in older men, and an estimated 10 to 12 million men experience impotence. Treatment options range from a simple adjustment in medication to surgical implantation of a penile prosthesis. Sexual function can almost always be restored, but many men with chronic erectile dysfunction never seek help. A sensitive nurse who has an understanding of sexual health can steer those who need help toward treatment. [3.1, 12.2]

<304> Power-Smith, P. (1991). **Problems in older people's longer term sexual relationships.** *Sexual and Marital Therapy, 6,* 287-296.

Discusses physical and sexual problems encountered by men and women in long-term relationships. Three relationship patterns frequently encountered in clinical practice presenting with unsatisfactory, infrequent, or no sexual contact are described, including too close, too distant, and too close/too distant polarization. Therapeutic approaches are presented. [3.1]

<305> Rowland, D. L., Greenleaf, W. J., Dorfman, L. J., & Davidson, J. M. (1993). **Aging and sexual function in men.** *Archives of Sexual Behavior, 22,* 545-557.

Attempts to identify sensory/neural and autonomic factors related to the decline of sexual function and erectile capacity in men as they age. Questionnaire data on sexual activity and functioning are gathered from 39 healthy, sexually functional men ages 21-82. Penile sensitivity, response to penile ischemia, and somatosensory evoked potentials show age-related changes. Significant age-related decreases occur in self-reported frequency of sexual activity and in erectile response to erotica. By contrast, self-reported erectile capacity, ratings of overall sex life, and levels of testosterone do not change over the age groups. The findings suggest that decreasing erectile capacity in aging men may be related to decreasing sensory/neural and autonomic functioning, but the findings also indicate factors other than the frequency and potency of sexual response are important to the overall rating of sex life. [3.1, 6.2]

<306> Schiavi, R. C. (1990). **Sexuality and aging in men.** *Annual Review of Sex Research, 1,* 227-249.

Critically reviews empirical literature on the sexuality of aging men with specific attention to issues of health and illness and age-related changes in sexual behavior. Discusses possible contributing factors to the variability among men. Reviews information on biological processes that may mediate the effect of aging in sexuality, and presents findings from an ongoing cross-sectional study of behavioral, hormonal, and psychological factors affecting the sexuality of healthy men (age 45-74 yrs) living in stable sexual relationships. Preliminary results show significant age-related declines in sexual desire, sexual arousal and activity, and erectile capacity but no differences in sexual or marital satisfaction. [3.1]

<307> Schiavi, R. C., Schreiner-Engel, P., Mandeli, J., Schanzer, H., & Cohen, E. (1990). **Healthy aging and male sexual function.** *American Journal of Psychiatry, 147,* 766-771.

Examines the effects of age on men's sexuality (sexual function and behavior) and on nocturnal penile tumescence in 65 healthy married men age 45-74. A significant negative relation exists between age and sexual desire, sexual arousal, and sexual activity, and there is an increasing prevalence of sexual dysfunction with age but no age difference in sexual enjoyment and satisfaction. Increasing age was also correlated with decreases in frequency, duration, and degree of nocturnal penile tumesence. [2.1, 3.1, 6.2]

<308> Vermeulen, A. (1991). Androgens in the aging male. *Journal of Clinical Endocrinology and Metabolism, 73,* 221-224.

Fertility persists into old age for men. Nevertheless old age in men is accompanied by clinical signs, such as a decrease in muscle and bone mass, decrease in sexual hair growth, and decrease libido and sexual activity, suggesting decreases in virility. The aging process is also accompanied by a significant decrease in bioavailable androgen levels, probably a consequence of a decreased Leydig cell mass and testicular perfusion. [2.1]

<309> Weiss, J. N., & Mellinger, B. C. (1990). Sexual dysfunction in elderly men. *Clinics In Geriatric Medicine, 6,* 185-196.

Reviews how the incidence of sexual dysfunction increases with age, and it argues how, in addition to normal physiologic changes of aging, the increased incidence of chronic disease and various medications affect sexual functioning. The authors discuss how sexual dysfunction should be investigated and treated in a manner acceptable to the patient. [2.1, 3.1, 6.2, 12.2]

SEXUAL LIFE

<310> Ade-Ridder, L. (1990). Sexuality and marital quality among older married couples. In T. H. Brubaker (Ed.), *Family relationships in later life* (pp. 48-67). Newbury Park, CA: Sage Publications.

Reviews current research findings about sexual behaviors and interests of older men and women as related to marital quality. Considers physiological aging factors that may influence sexual functioning, as well as the reported behaviors and interests expressed by the older persons who have participated in the small number of research studies. Original data are presented for 488 married older men and women about their sexual interests and behaviors. [2.1, 3.2, 6.2, 8.4]

<311> Antonovsky, H., Sadowsky, M., & Maoz, B. (1990). Sexual activity of aging men and women: An Israeli study. *Behavior, Health, and Aging, 1,* 151-161.

Too few investigations examine the sexual behavior of aging men and women. This study provides basic information on sexual activity, interest, satisfaction in the present and the in past, and attitudes about sexuality for 177 older men and 122 women age 65-85 living in Israel in private dwellings. The most important factors accounting for sexual activity in aging men are sexual desire, marital status, and health. Although age is related to sexual behavior, its impact is less important than most of the other variables studied. At the interview, two-thirds of the women and one-third of the men report that they had ceased having sexual intercourse. Of women, 12 percent stopped because their husbands are impotent, and 64 percent stopped because of the death of their husbands. Of men, 29 percent stopped intercourse because of their own health problems, and 24 percent stopped because of the death of their wives. [3.2, 8.4]

<312> Bastida, E. (1987). **Sex-typed age norms among older Hispanics.** *The Gerontologist*, 27, 59-65.

Hypothesizes that age norms vary with class, gender, and ethnicity, and examines the age identification and importance of gender-specific, age-appropriate behavior among 160 older Hispanics of Mexican, Puerto Rican, and Cuban origin. Content analysis of the open ended questions in structured interviews finds men and women from all three ethnic groups use realistic age norms when discussing self-expectations. When addressing sexuality and what is consider appropriate behavior, there is congruence with traditional gender socialization. Sexuality is accepted among elders, and there are fewer sanctioned norms for men than for women. [3.2]

<313> Bergstrom, W., Maj, B., & Nielsen, H. H. (1990). **Sexual expression among 60-80-year-old men and women: A sample from Stockholm, Sweden.** *Journal of Sex Research*, 27, 289-295.

Investigates sexual interests and activity (masturbation, sexual intercourse), and physical and mental health of 509 men and women age 60-80 from Stockholm. Sexual interest and activity are routinely present--61 percent of the elder group expressed their sexuality through intercourse, mutual sexual stimulation, and masturbation. Men are significantly more sexual than women, in all ages and in all respects. Sexual interest and activity significantly decrease in ages 75-80, albeit nearly one-quarter of the elders have intercourse at least sometime each month. [3.2]

<314> Bretschneider, J. G., & McCoy, N. L. (1988). **Sexual interest and behavior in healthy 80- to 102-year-olds.** *Archives of Sexual Behavior*, 17, 109-129.

Studies the sexual interest and behavior of 100 healthy, upper middle-class white men and 102 women living in residential retirement facilities. Finds the most common activity was touching and caressing without sexual intercourse, followed by masturbation, then sexual intercourse. Only touching and caressing show significant decline from the 80s to the 90s, with the decline in this activity for men but not for women. With two exceptions (past enjoyment of sexual intercourse and enjoyment of touching and caressing without sexual intercourse), reports reflect more activity and enjoyment by men. Except for frequency of sexual intercourse, the correlation between past and present frequency of sexual behaviors are substantial, suggesting that current physical and social factors have an overriding role in this area. [1.1, 3.2]

<315> Butler, R. N., & Lewis, M. I. (1976). *Sex after sixty: A guide for men and women for their later years.* **New York: Harper and Row.**

A seminal book written for older men and women who are interested in sex and for people who want to understand elders better. Presents a number of possible solutions to sexual problems, and proposes means for countering negative attitudes that older people may experience--within themselves, from family members, from the medical and psychotherapeutic professions, and from society at large. Recognizes that even individuals who have a lively enthusiasm and capacity for sex need information, support, and sometimes various kinds of treatment in order to continue sexual activity. Chapters focus on normal physical changes in sex and sexuality with age, common medical and emotional problems with sex, learning new patterns of lovemaking, dating and remarriage, and where to find outside professional help. [3.2]

<316> Cogen, R., & Steinman, W. (1990). Sexual function and practice in elderly men of lower socioeconomic status. *Journal of Family Practice, 31*, 162-166.

Determines the prevalence of erectile dysfunction and examines the sexual practices and attitudes of 87 men age 60 and older from predominantly blue-collar backgrounds. Slightly more than one in four men report complete loss of erectile function, and another 31 percent report frequent difficulties achieving vaginal intromission.   Unlike economically advantaged groups' decisions to continue sexual activity by alternative practices, only 29 percent used mutual masturbation and 16 percent used oral sex. Attitudes toward these practices were negative. Men unable to perform coitus ceased heterosexual activity. [3.2, 8.4]

<317> Covey, H. C. (1989). Perceptions and attitudes toward sexuality of the elderly during the middle ages. *The Gerontologist, 29*, 93-100.

Identifies in literature, art, and historical works major themes from the European Middle Ages regarding sexuality and aging. Conceptions of aging excluded the elderly from having normal sex lives, and the church of the Middle Ages defined sexual behavior by elders as immoral. Medieval physiological theories hold that sexual decline occurs much more dramatically and earlier for women than men, however older men's sex lives are not clearly defined. Older men attempting to maintain sex lives were typically ridiculed, nonetheless sexual activity was commonly thought to prolong their life. [3.2, 6.2]

<318> Creti, L., & Libman E. (1989). Cognitions and sexual expression in the aging. *Journal of Sex and Marital Therapy, 15*, 83-101.

Investigates the sexual frequency, desired sexual frequency, and quality of sexual functioning in aging couples where the male had undergone transurethral prostatectomy. Data are from 32 married couples (age 50-77). Finds in this sample of sexually active couples, high sexual efficacy expectations predict high couple sexual frequency and good male and female sexual functioning. High individual sexual drive predict high actual and desired couple sexual interaction.   In general, it is the male's sexual confidence and drive that is highly related to couple sexual expression. [3.2, 12.2]

<319> Keil, J. E., Sutherland, S. E., Knapp, R. G., Waid, L. R., & Gazes, P. C. (1992). Self-reported sexual functioning in elderly blacks and whites. *Journal of Aging and Health, 4,* 112-125.

Examines problems of sexual arousal and activity among the survivors of the Charleston Heart Study cohort age 60 and older. Nearly 50 percent report problems with becoming sexually aroused. Whether having a physiological or psychological basis, problems diminish frequency of coital activity. By comparison, 41 percent of white men and 37 percent of black men age 80 and older report no problems with arousal. Age and arousal status are highly related to each other and to sexual frequency. Other predictors of arousal problems are physical disability, increased use of prescription drugs, lower pulmonary function, and self-rated health as poor. Correlates of sexual frequency vary for each sex and race subgroup. [3.2]

<320> Litz, B. T., Zeiss, A. M., & Davies, H. D. (1990). Sexual concerns of male spouses of female Alzheimer's disease patients. *The Gerontologist, 30,* 113-116.

Discusses how dementia presents a caregiver with many, often conflicting challenges to sexual functioning. A case study highlights issues of conflict between husbands and their Alzheimer's-effected wives. The case describes a man who reports erectile dysfunction directly stemming from stressful changes that had occurred in his relationship to his wife who had Alzheimer's disease. General themes and relevant hypotheses are derived and clinical practice implications are explored. [3.2, 8.4, 9.1]

<321> Marsiglio, W., & Donnelly, D. (1991). Sexual relations in later life: A national study of married persons. *Journals of Gerontology: Social Sciences, 46,* S338-S344.

Using the National Survey of Families and Households, examines the sexual behavior among married persons age 60 and older. About 53 percent of the entire sample, and about 24 percent of those age 76 and older report having sexual relations at least once within the past month. A sense of self-worth and competence, marital satisfaction, and the spouse's health status are positively related to the incidence of sexual relations within the past month, and age is negatively related to monthly incidence and overall sexual frequency. Gender or a gender-by-spouse's health status interaction term were not related to sexual behavior within the context of marriage and long-term coupled relationships. [3.2, 8.4]

<322> Marsiglio, W., & Greer, R. A. (1994). A gender analysis of older men's sexuality: Social, psychological and biological dimensions. In E. Thompson (Ed.), *Older men's lives* (pp. 122-140). Thousand Oaks, CA: Sage Publications.

Theorizes that older men's sexual self-concept and sexual behavior are affected primarily by cultural and sexual scenarios, previous sexual experience and attitudes, and the physiological changes associated with aging. Reviews how sexual scripts within traditional masculinity ideology affect the way older men experience their sexuality and the way others perceive older men, and underscores how men's sexuality cannot be understood outside its gendered, sociocultural context. Although physiological aging does have a profound impact on sexual experiences, concludes that the social and psychological dimensions of sexuality influence adaptation to aging and men's sexuality in later-life. [3.2, 6.2]

<323> **Martin, C. E. (1981). Factors affecting sexual functioning in 60-70 year-old married males.** *Archives of Sexual Behavior*, **10, 399-420.**

In data from the Baltimore Longitudinal Study of Aging, finds former levels of sexual functioning significantly correlated with current functioning, supporting hypothesis that men generally maintain relatively high or low rates of sexual activity throughout their lives. The frequency of sexual expression was also independent of such factors as marital adjustment, sexual attractiveness of wives, sexual attitudes, and demographic features of marital history. By comparison, sexual frequency, erotic response to visual stimuli, and time comfortable without sex are closely related, suggesting the importance of motivation. [3.1]

<324> **Persson, G., & Svanborg, A. (1992). Marital coital activity in men at the age of 75: Relation to somatic, psychiatric, and social factors at the age of 70.** *Journal of the American Geriatrics Society*, **40, 439-444.**

What predicts cessation of coital activity in elderly married men. Interviews with 41 men who are married and had coital activity at age 70 and who, at the age of 75 are still married, reveals the prevalence of coital activity decreases from about 50 percent at the age of 70 to about 30 percent at the age of 75. Cessation of coital activity is associated with vasculogenic factors, such as systemic hypertension and ischemic heart disease, and types of stress experienced between age 65 and 70, but there is no association with any psychiatric or social factor. Knowing cardiovascular disorders are associated with aging strongly suggests that aging in itself has an impact on sexual performance in the age interval studied. [2.1, 3.2, 8.4]

<325> **Pope, M., & Schulz, R. (1990). Sexual attitudes and behavior in midlife and aging homosexual males.** *Journal of Homosexuality*, **20, 169-177.**

Describes older gay men's self-reports of sexual attitudes and behavior. The data are from 87 homosexual men age 40-77 in the Chicago area. The primary finding is that the majority are currently sexually active and want to remain sexually involved. Concludes that older gay men maintain both their interest in sex and their ability to function sexually. [3.2]

<326> **Schiavi, R. C., Mandeli, J., & Schreiner-Engel, P. (1994). Sexual satisfaction in healthy aging men.** *Journal Sex and Marital Therapy*, **20, 3-13.**

Systematic information on what contributes to sexual satisfaction in healthy older men is lacking. This study explores the predictive significance of psychological, marital, and behavioral variables and their interaction on the satisfaction of healthy married volunteers age 45 to 74. Subjects' perception of erectile difficulties, sexual information, affect, and marital adjustment have differential correlations with three measures of sexual satisfaction. The authors review how these results mark the need to move beyond an exclusive focus on performance to the determinants of sexual enjoyment and satisfaction in the later years. [3.2]

<327> Thomas, L. E. (1991). Correlates of sexual interest among elderly men. *Psychological Reports, 68*, 620-622.

Interviews from 46 English elderly men (age 70 to 94 years) tap sexual attitudes, psychological traits, and life satisfaction. Sexual interest is correlated with measures of emotional expressivity, personal identity, as well as regrets about the past, but not with marital status nor life satisfaction. Findings are discussed in terms of Erikson's later stages of ego development. [1.5, 3.2]

<328> Weizman, R., & Hart, J. (1987). Sexual behavior in healthy married elderly men. *Archives of Sexual Behavior, 16*, 39-44.

Evaluates the sexual behavior in 81 married men age 60-71 using self-report rating scales. More than one-third (36 percent) report experiencing impotence, and about half of the men report regular masturbatory activity. Frequency of sexual intercourse declines and frequency of masturbation increases among the 47 older men age 66-71 compared to the 34 younger men age 60-65. These data indicate that the interest in sexuality continues in elderly men, although the form of sexual expression changes from active sexual intercourse to a self-pleasuring/autoerotic form. [3.2]

<329> Whitebourne, S. K. (1990). Sexuality in the aging male. *Generations, 14* (3), 28-30.

Reviews the effect of aging on the men's sexuality. Men in their late 60s and 70s do not experience a distinct climacteric phase during which they lose reproductive capacity, rather they experience a gradual loss of the quantity of viable sperm. More noticeable to the aging male are a variety of changes in the prostate gland, the rhythmic contractions of which contribute to the sensation of orgasm. Research has also found that older men experience a general slowing down of the progression through the phases of the human sexual response cycle, from excitement through resolution. The literature suggests that men's pattern of sexuality in earlier years is the best predictor of their sexuality in old age. [3.2]

4

Suicide and Alcohol

— ◆ —

SUICIDE

<330> Blazer, D. G. (1991). Suicide risk factors in the elderly: An empirical study. *Journal of Geriatric Psychiatry, 24*, 175-189.

Reports on the well established relationship between old age and suicide, but the less well known risk factors. Proposes that gender is a risk factor which interacts with age. Older males commit suicide at a higher rate than any other age by gender group. The association between suicide and age can be explained almost exclusively by elderly men's suicide. Concludes that the relative difference in suicide rates between older men and women has remained fairly constant during the latter part of the century. [4.1]

<331> Canetto, S. S. (1992). Gender and suicide in the elderly. *Suicide and Life Threatening Behavior, 22*, 80-97.

Discusses explanations for the comparatively high rates of suicide mortality among elderly men and low rates among elderly women. Social and economic factors do not appear to account for men's lack of "resilience," but there are indications of gender differences in coping. Men are less flexible in responses and have fewer coping strategies available. Socialization seems to impact on suicides through definitions of gender-appropriate suicides. Evidence suggests suicidal death in older men is rein-forced by masculinity ideology's emphasis on lethal suicide. Older men may anticipate being ridiculed and disliked if they survive suicide. Suggests prevention should focus on gender socialization experiences and roles. It is likely that experiences and respon-sibilities as part of relationships are the key to suicide prevention among older men. [1.4, 4.1]

<332> Glass, J. C. Jr., & Reed, S. E. (1993). To live or die: A look at elderly suicide. *Educational Gerontology, 19*, 767-778.

Reviews the characteristics of late-life suicides and discusses strategies for intervention. The elderly are at higher risk for suicide than any other age group, and elderly suicide is significantly underreported. Some of the characteristics of this high-risk population are a genuine wish to die, the use of more lethal methods than younger persons use, and generally poorer physical health. Elderly white men, especially widowers, are the group at highest risk for suicide, and elderly nonwhites have lower suicide rates than elderly whites. Practitioners working with elderly persons are urged to recognize the clues that indicate suicidal behavior, evaluate the degree of risk for a successful suicide attempt, and carry out appropriate interventions. Ten suggested strategies for lowering the elderly suicide rate are provided. [4.1]

<333> Horton-Deutsch, S. L., Clark, D. C., & Farran, C. J. (1992). Chronic dyspnea and suicide in elderly men. *Hospital and Community Psychiatry*, *43*, 1198-1203.

Explores links between chronic dyspnea and suicide risk among elderly men, by retrospectively examining the charts of 14 men age 65-93 who expressed concern about their inability to breathe in the weeks or months before their suicides. They had at least one of three illnesses associated with chronic dyspnea--chronic obstructive pulmonary disease, congestive heart failure, and lung cancer. Spouses, children, or siblings of the deceased are interviewed about circumstances of the suicide, mental status in the week prior to death, and lifetime history of psychiatric disorders. All 14 men suffered from some type of depressive illness, and 13 of the 14 experienced the loss of a loved one after a period of suffering. All are described as proud, rigid men who had difficulty accepting help from others. Recommends that clinicians evaluate patients for their perceptions and psychological responses, and those at risk be referred for treatment. [2.2, 4.1, 12.2]

<334> Kaplan, M. S., Adamek, M. E., & Johnson, S. (1994). Trends in firearm suicide among older American males: 1979-1988. *The Gerontologist*, *34*, 59-65.

Performs age-specific analysis of men's suicide trends. Elderly men are more likely to commit suicide than any other age group in the United States, and their rate steadily increased between 1979 and 1988. Men age 65 and older are most likely to use firearms, followed by those 55-64. In 1988, nearly 8 out of 10 suicides by men age 65 and older were committed with a firearm. Of the 43,159 suicides by elder men during the 10-year period, nearly three out of four are firearm-related. Firearm-related suicides are much lower for elderly blacks than whites, however the rate of undetermined death for black men is 213 percent higher than for whites, suggesting blacks suicide rates must be interpreted with caution. [4.1]

<335> Lindesay, J. (1991). Suicide in the elderly. *International Journal of Geriatric Psychiatry*, *6*, 355-361.

Reviews research that may aid in understanding suicide in elderly persons in the United Kingdom. Suggests that there has been little change in the overall rates of suicide in this population over the past decade. However, analgesics are now the most common drugs of suicide, and there has been a steady increase in suicides by car exhausts in elderly men. Addresses the issue of suicide prevention, and notes that even in the terminally ill elderly person, suicidal thoughts are associated with depression and respond to treatment. [4.1]

<336> McCall, P. L. (1991). Adolescent and elderly white male suicide trends:

Evidence of changing well-being? *Journals of Gerontology: Social Sciences, 46,* S43-S51.

Age- and sex-specific suicide rates exhibit different patterns over the life course. Since World War II, elderly men's suicide rates declined as adolescent boys' rates increased, and the most dramatic shifts are noted among whites. Investigates the relationship proposed by Preston between suicide and the changing status of America's dependent populations -- that is, adolescents' declining well-being and elder's improving well-being. Findings do suggest that family dissolution and living in poverty are associated with white adolescents' suicide trends, whereas societal affluence is linked to white elderly men's trends. [4.1]

<337> Rich, C. L., Warstadt, G. M., Nemiroff, R. A., Fowler, R. C., Young, D., & Warstadt, G. M. (1991). Suicide, stressors, and the life cycle. *American Journal of Psychiatry, 48,* 524-527.

Examines relationships between stressors, suicide, and stages of the life cycle. Using the initial 204 consecutive cases from the San Diego Suicide Study, information is gathered from family members, spouses, acquaintances, employers, other witnesses, physicians, and other professionals. Predictable patterns are noted for the three most common stressor groups: conflict-separation-rejection, economic problems, and medical illness. The only gender difference is that more men than women have economic problems as a stressor, and the majority of the stressors among subjects 80 years or older are illnesses. The variations in the patterns of stressors found in this study of suicides coincide with adult development theory. [1.5, 4.1]

ALCOHOL

<338> Atkinson, R, M., Tolson, R. L., & Turner, J. A. (1990). Late versus early onset problem drinking in older men. *Alcoholism: Clinical and Experimental Research, 14,* 574-579.

Age at onset of problem drinking was studied in 132 men age 60 and older who were admitted to a Veterans Administration geriatric alcoholism outpatient treatment program. Examines demographics, alcohol history, self-reported psychological status, special treatment, and treatment compliance variables for association with onset age. Late onset (defined as onset at or after age 60) is not uncommon, occurring in 15% of the sample and 29% of patients age 65 or older. Compared to earlier onset cases, late onset alcohol problems are milder, more circumscribed, associated with less family alcoholism, and greater psychological stability. Late onset patients are also more compliant with outpatient treatment requirements. [4.2]

<339> Black, S. A., & Markides, K. S. (1994). Aging and generational patterns of alcohol consumption among Mexican Americans, Cuban Americans, and mainland Puerto Ricans. *International Journal of Aging and Human Development, 39,* 97-103.

Describes the life-course patterns of alcohol comsumption among 2,827 Mexican Amercians, 799 Cuban Americans, and 1,043 Puerto Ricans, all age 25-74 and residing in the mainland U.S. Data are from the Hispanic Health and Nutrition Examination Survey. Consumption among Mexican Americans and Puerto Ricans is found to have aging effects, as evidenced by increasing percentages of former drinkers coupled with consistently low percentages of abstainers at all ages. However, among Cuban Americans, cohort effects are more evident for middle-age and older men, since they continue their low consumption rates from younger years. [4.2]

<340> Brennan, P. L., & Moos, R. H. (1990). Life stressors, social resources, and late-life problem drinking. *Psychology and Aging, 5*, 491-501.

Studies life stressors and social resources among late-middle-aged problem (N = 501) and nonproblem drinkers (N = 609). Problem drinkers report more negative life events, chronic stressors, and social resource deficits. Among problem drinkers, men report more ongoing stressors involving chronic financial difficulties and problems with friends, and less support from children, kin, and friends than women. Lack of support and presence of stressors may be overlapping. [2.3, 4.2, 7.5]

<341> Chaikelson, J. S., Arbuckle, T. Y., Lapidus, S., & Gold, D. P. (1994). Measurement of lifetime alcohol consumption. *Journal of Studies on Alcohol, 55*, 133-140.

Examines the interdependent assumptions that social drinking behavior is highly consistent across the life span, and that assessment in a particular period is a reliable indicator of individual's normal drinking. Patterns of lifetime drinking reveal a decline in drinking beginning on average about 55 years of age. Validity of these reports are tested with each wife's rating, and her ratings confirm. [4.2]

<342> Colsher, P. L., & Wallace, R. B. (1990). Elderly men with histories of heavy drinking: Correlates and consequences. *Journal of Studies on Alcohol, 51*, 528-535.

Studies the impact of lifetime drinking habits of 1,155 older men, and examines the characteristics of men with self-reported histories of heavy drinkers. Data are from a longitudinal survey of community-based elders. Ten percent of the men report that they had been heavy drinkers at some time during their lives. They are less educated, have higher mortality, and report more major illnesses, poorer self-perceived health, lower life satisfaction, and smaller social networks. A history of having been a heavy drinker is predictive of widespread impairments in physical, psychological, and social health and functioning. [2.1, 4.2]

<343> Ekerdt, D. J., De Labry, L. O., Glynn, R. J., & Davis, R. W. (1989). Change in drinking behaviors with retirement: Findings from the Normative Aging Study. *Journal of Studies on Alcohol, 50*, 347-353.

Recognizes that retirement can be a dysphoric experience and unstructured time creates greater opportunity for alcohol consumption. Examines changes in drinking behavior over an approximately 2-year span in two groups of community-dwelling men, recently retired and still employed. Results indicate that retirement is not a predictor of changes in average alcohol consumption, although retirees show greater variability over the two years. Although change of routine has the potential for being disruptive, retirement does not have a deleterious effect on drinking behavior. [4.2, 10.2]

<344> Jennison, K. M. (1992). The impact of stressful live events and social support on drinking among older adults: A general population survey. *International Journal of Aging and Human Development, 35,* 99-123.

Analyzes the importance of stressful life events and the buffering hypothesis to alcohol use in a national sample of 1,418 men and women age 60 and older. Excessive drinking among elders, as with drinking in general, is disproportionately a male activity and is more common among never- and formerly-married men. Elders who have stressful losses are significantly more likely to drink excessively than those who have not experienced these losses. Alcohol use may represent an attempt to cope with traumatic loss. Drinking is reported to increase during periods of prolonged exposure to emotionally depleting life change and loss. Supportive resources of spouse, family, friends, and church do have stress buffering effects, yet traumatic losses within these networks coupled with supportive needs may exceed the resources. [4.2, 7.5]

<345> Krause, N. (1991). Stress, religiosity, and abstinence from alcohol. *Psychology and Aging, 6,* 134-144.

Tests a model designed to identify psychosocial factors associated with the avoidance of alcohol in later life. The premise is that certain stressors (e.g., health problems, financial difficulties) may be related to abstinence from alcohol. The effects of a potentially important coping resource (religiosity) are included to specify the relationship between stress and abstinence more accurately. Finds within data from the Americans' Changing Lives Survey that older adults who abstain from alcohol report fewer health problems. As health problems increase, elders who report greater subjective religious involvement and, in turn, report more abstinence from alcohol. Gender has a marked effect on each construct (e.g., men (and women) with greater religiousness more likely abstain from alcohol in later life). However, because men tend to have less religious involvement, abstinence from alcohol in later life is noteworthy. [2.3, 4.2, 5.1]

<346> Liberto, J. G., Oslin, D. W., & Ruskin, P. E. (1992). Alcoholism in older persons: A review of the literature. *Hospital and Community Psychiatry, 43,* 975-984.

Reviews patterns of alcohol abuse and dependence in the elderly. The most consistent finding of cross-sectional and longitudinal studies demonstrates the quantity and frequency of alcohol consumption are higher in elderly men than in elderly women, as is the prevalence of alcohol-related problems. Elderly persons with lower incomes consume less alcohol than those with higher incomes. Both hospitalized and outpatient populations have more problem drinkers, and the elderly alcoholic is at greater risk for medical and psychiatric comorbidity. About one-third to one-half of elderly alcoholics experience the onset of problem drinking in middle or late life. Outcomes seem to be better for those who have late-onset drinking. [4.2, 12.2]

<347> Lopez-Bushnell, F. K., Tyra, P. A., & Futrell, M. (1992). Alcoholism and the Hispanic older adult. *Clinical Gerontologist, 11* (3/4), 123-130.

Discusses how in the Hispanic culture, drinking patterns vary with gender and how alcoholism is part of elders' lives. Thirteen percent of older men report frequent drinking, while only 3% of women report such behavior. These patterns are contextualized as cultural factors and men's gendered perceptions of health. [4.2]

<348> Moos, R. H., Brennan, P. L., Fondacaro, M. R., & Moos, B. S. (1990). Approach and avoidance coping responses among older problem and non-problem drinkers. *Psychology and Aging, 5,* 31-40.

The Coping Response Inventory organizes coping efforts according to their focus (approach or avoidance) and method (cognitive or behavioral). Compared with non-problem drinkers, older problem drinkers are more likely to use cognitive and behavioral avoidance to manage life stressors. Problem drinking men report more negative life events and are less likely to seek guidance and support than nonproblem drinking men, who are more likely married and have a coresident confidant. [4.2]

<349> Rivers, P. C., Rivers, L. S., & Newman, D. L. (1991). Alcohol and aging: A cross-gender comparison. *Psychology of Addictive Behaviors, 5,* 41-47.

Examines measures of psychosocial functioning for alcoholic and nonalcoholic men (N=60) and women (N=57) age 55 and older. Measures include the Michigan Alcoholism Screening Test (MAST), the Heimler Scale of Social Functioning (HSSF), and several scales from the Scheidt-Windley (S-W) study of rural elderly. Men who are alcoholics have show more severe psychopathology on the MAST. [4.2]

<350> Seymour, J., & Wattis, J. P. (1992). Alcohol abuse in the elderly. *Reviews in Clinical Gerontology, 2* (2), 141-150.

Discusses the way definitions of alcohol abuse and dependence are applied to older people, reviews the effects of aging on alcohol metabolism, and presents the epidemiology and the causes of alcohol abuse in old age. Concludes that alcohol abuse is relatively common in the 65-75 age range but less common in very old people. Alcohol dependence, strictly defined, is rare. Alcohol abuse in elderly men and particularly women is under-recognized by primary care workers and hospital doctors, as the presentation is often nonspecific. [4.2]

5

Religion and Spirituality

— ◆ —

RELIGION AND RELIGIOSITY

<351> Blazer, D. G., & Palmore, E. B. (1976). Religion and aging in a longitudinal panel. *The Gerontologist, 16,* 82-85.

Shows that religious behaviors are more important than religious attitudes to feelings of usefulness, happiness, and adjustment, especially for men over 70 and men from manual labor backgrounds. [2.3, 5.1]

<352> Chatters, L. M., & Taylor, R. J. (1989). Age differences in religious participation among black adults. *Journals of Gerontology: Social Sciences, 44,* S183-S189.

Determines age differences in level of religious participation using data from 2,107 black Americans age 18 and older. Examines seven indicators of organizational, nonorganizational, and attitudinal forms of religious involvement. For men, request for prayer from others is the only measure for which age was not a predictor; among women, age is positively associated with each measure. Concludes that black adults seem to manifest high levels of organized religious participation as well as involvement in private, non-organizational religious pursuits. [5.1]

<353> Courtenay, B. C., Poon, L. W., Martin, P., Clayton, G. M., & Johnson, M. A. (1992). Religiosity and adaptation in the oldest-old. *International Journal of Aging & Human Development, 34,* 47-56.

Notes the equivocal results in prior work regarding the relationship between religiosity and adaptation in older adults. Although many studies believe religiosity is stable over the life span, religiosity may or may not be related to such factors as physical and mental health, life satisfaction, and coping. Determines that religiosity does not change significantly as one ages, that some relationship exists between religiosity and physical health, but no meaningful relationship is evident for religiosity and mental health or life satisfaction. Questions whether religious coping mechanisms are important among the oldest-old. [1.5, 5.1]

<354> Guy, R. F. (1982). Religion, physical disabilities, and life satisfaction in older age cohorts. *International Journal of Aging and Human Development, 15*, 225-232.

Examines the role of religion in the personal adjustment of older age cohorts, with emphasis on life satisfaction as it relates to age, physical disabilities, and church attendance. Data on 1,170 persons 60 years of age and older reveal positive findings on the relationship between religious activity and life satisfaction. Individuals attending church weekly scored highest on life satisfaction; and individuals with some physical limitations who attended infrequently scored higher on life satisfaction if some form of church contact (newsletters, telephone, personal visits) was maintained. [2.3, 5.1]

<355> Holt, M. K., & Dellmann-Jenkins, M. (1992). Research and implications for practice: Religion, well-being/morale, and coping behavior in later life. *Journal of Applied Gerontology, 11*, 101-110.

Reviews the importance of religion to older persons and the potential of religion as a resource for improving elders' quality of life. The multidimensional nature of religiosity and the role of religion in morale/well-being and coping are discussed. [2.3, 5.1]

<356> Idler, E. L. (1987). Religious involvement and the health of the elderly: Some hypotheses and an initial test. *Social Forces, 66*, 226-238.

Examines relationship between religious involvement and health. Data are from the Yale Health and Aging Project (N = 2811). Observes involvement is associated with lower levels of functional disability and depressive symptomalogy. The relationship between men's religiousness and health status is not accounted for by people's health behavior. At any given level of chronic illness, men who receive a great deal of comfort from religion report less disability and less depression. [2.2, 5.1]

<357> Idler, E. L., & Kasl, S. V. (1992). Religion, disability, depression, and the timing of death. *American Journal of Sociology, 97*, 1052-1079.

Examines longitudinally the relationship between religious involvement and health status in 2,812 men and women age 65 and older living in New Haven, Connecticut. There is a significant protective effect of public religious involvement against disability among both men and women, and of private religious involvement against depression among recently disabled men. Religious group membership protects Christians and Jews against mortality in the month before their respective religious holidays. Concludes that religious involvement exerts a strong positive effect on the health and this effect varies by religious group and gender. The health behaviors, social contacts, and optimistic attitudes of religious group members may explain part, but not all, of this association. [2.2, 5.1]

<358> Koenig, H. G. (1988). Religious behaviors and death anxiety in later life. *Hospice Journal, 4*, 3-24.

Examines the relationship between personal and community religious behaviors and feelings and the fear of death for 296 adults age 60 and older. Seven of eight elders express little or no fear of death. Those who are afraid employ religious beliefs and prayer during stressful situations. Those age 75+ are significantly more likely than "tepid" believers to report low or no fear about death. These cognitive coping behaviors may have relevance for sick and disabled older persons with few coping resources and little control over the environment. [2.3, 5.1]

<359> **Koenig, H. G. (1990). Research on religion and mental health in later life: A review and commentary.** *Journal of Geriatric Psychiatry, 23,* 23-53.

Discusses the efforts of recent cross-sectional and longitudinal studies to understand the relationships religiosity has with elders' mental health, functional disability, satisfaction with health, and perception of pain. Presents a range of implications of these findings for the clinical therapist. [2.1, 2.2, 5.1]

<360> **Koenig, H. G., Moberg, D. O., & Kvale, J. N. (1988). Religious activities and attitudes of older adults in a geriatric assessment clinic.** *Journal of the American Geriatrics Society, 36,* 362-374.

Studies the religiosity of 106 elderly adult patients age 56-94 attending a geriatric out-patient clinic. A high prevalence of orthodox Christian beliefs, religious community ac-tivity, private devotional activity is observed. Intrinsic religiosity is lower among men with hypertension. Religious activity is lower for those with cancer, chronic anxiety, and depressive symptoms. Religion seems to be a powerful cultural force in the lives of older medical patients, related to both mental and physical health. [2.1, 2.2, 5.1]

<361> **Krause, N., & Van Tran, T. (1989). Stress and religious involvement among older blacks.** *Journals of Gerontology: Social Sciences, 44,* S4-S13.

Determines whether religious involvement helps to reduce the negative impact of stressful life events (as measured by self-esteem and feelings of personal control) in a nationwide sample of older blacks. Evaluating three models of the stress process--the suppressor, moderator, and distress-deterrent--finds the distress-deterrent model best fits older blacks' experiences. Gender is not directly predictive of differences in outcomes; however, religious involvement reduces the effects of stress and men have lower involvement than women. [2.3, 5.1]

<362> **Levin, J. S. (1988). Religious factors in aging, adjustment, and health: A theoretical overview.** *Journal of Religion & Aging, 4,* 133-146.

Reviews six theoretical viewpoints which have guided gerontological research on religion and health: activity theory, a "deterioration" perspective, the social decrement or isolation model, disengagement theory, an "eschatological" perspective, and the multidimensional disengagement perspective of Mindel and Vaughan. [2.2, 5.1]

<363> **Levin, J. S., & Taylor, R. J. (1993). Gender and age differences in religios-ity among black Americans.** *The Gerontologist, 33,* 16-23.

Examines gender and age differences over a dozen indicators of religiosity. Uses the National Survey of Black Americans (N = 2107). Religiosity is greater in successive ages among black men, with older men very actively involved in religion. Perhaps black men become more religious with age relative to black women. Despite closing the gender gap, it persists--black men remain less religious than black women. [5.1]

<364> Levin, J. S., Taylor, R. J., & Chatters, L. M. (1994). Race and gender differ-
ences in religiosity among older adults: Findings from four national
surveys. *Journals of Gerontology: Social Sciences, 49*, S137-S145.

Using data from the second Quality of American Life survey, the Myth and Realities of
Aging study, the first wave of Americans' Changing Lives, and the 1987 sample of the
General Social Survey, this article examines racial and gender patterns within elders'
religiosity. In all four studies, whites and men report less religiosity. Of 21 comparisons
with indicators of religiosity, gender differences are noted on 13, and older men are less
religious on each. Blacks are more religious on 19 of the 21, and black men display
higher levels of religious involvement than older white women on all but four
comparisons. [5.1]

<365> Markides, K. S., Levin, J. S., & Ray, L. A. (1987). Religion, aging, and life
satisfaction: An eight-year, three-wave longitudinal study. *The Gerontologist, 27*, 660-665.

Challenges common assumptions that there is evidence that older men or women
increasingly turn to religion as they age, decline in health, and approach death. Data
from a three-wave longitudinal study of older Mexican-Americans and some Anglos
demonstrate that indicators of religiosity, with exception of religious attendance, remain
fairly stable over time. Religiosity is not predictive of life satisfaction. [2.3, 5.1]

<366> Morse, C. K., & Wisocki, P. A. (1987). Importance of religiosity to elderly
adjustment. *Journal of Religion & Aging, 4*, 15-26.

Religious beliefs and practices have long been considered as important to psychological
adjustment and in the lives of older people. Finds in a sample of 156 elders (age 60-90)
from senior center programs that neither age nor gender is correlated with religiosity;
however elders with higher levels of religious activity and belief are more psychologically
healthy and more socially involved. [2.2, 5.1]

<367> Nelson, P. B. (1989). Ethnic differences in intrinsic/extrinsic religious
orientation and depression in the elderly. *Archives of Psychiatric Nursing,
3*, 199-204.

Comparative analysis of religious participation of black and white elderly individuals
indicates that religion is important for both groups, however black and white elders differ
in religious behavior and the role that religion plays in coping with the adversities of
aging. Although black elders are more intrinsically oriented to religion than are white
elders, and more depressed than are whites, correlations show a negative relationship
between intrinsic religious orientation and depression. [2.3, 5.1]

<368> Nye, W. P. (1992-93). Amazing grace: Religion and identity among elderly
black individuals. *International Journal of Aging and Human Development,
36*, 103-114.

Investigates the fit of continuity theory to aging among African-Americans. The data are

43 "life stories" from middle-class African-American men and women who range in age from 56 to 94. Listening for the "themes" presented within and across life stories, examines the importance of the "theme" religion has as a bulwark of continuity in the lives of the respondents. Finds religion does serve a number of significant and positive purposes in the normal aging of black Americans, perhaps more than the continuity provided by kinship or the self-building functions of work. [5.1]

<369> Rosik, C. H. (1989). The impact of religious orientation in conjugal bereavement among older adults. *International Journal of Aging and Human Development, 28,* 251-260.

With a sample of 159 elderly widowed, examines the relationship between religious commitment and adaptation to widowhood. Widowers mild depression and grief remain, while widows depression level returns to normal about five to seven years after the death of the spouse. Greater religiosity, especially when oriented toward gaining support and comfort, is significantly associated with distress, particularly for the widowers. [2.3, 5.1]

<370> Taylor, R. J. (1986). Religious participation among elderly blacks. *The Gerontologist, 26,* 630-636.

Studies three indicators of religious participation among elder blacks: frequency of religious service attendance, church membership, and the degree of subjective religiosity. Finds the elder black men participate less than elder women. Religious participation also varied by marital status, age, and urban residence. Despite level of participation, religion and the church are important aspects of the lives of elderly black men. The importance of religion and the church for social service agencies is discussed. [5.1]

<371> Taylor, R. J., & Chatters, L. M. (1991). Nonorganizational religious participation among elderly black adults. *Journals of Gerontology: Social Sciences, 46,* S103-S111.

Describes four areas of religious activity--reading religious materials, watching or listening to religious programs, prayer, and requests for prayer--for 366 female and 215 male elderly blacks, age 55-101. Gender is the strongest and most consistent predictor, with men reporting less participation. Health, other demographics, and religious denomination influence religiosity. A majority of men report they pray daily, read religious materials, watch or listen to religious programs on a weekly basis, and request prayer on their own behalf several times per month. [5.1]

<372> Thorson, J. A., & Powell, F. C. (1989). Death anxiety and religion in an older male sample. *Psychological Reports, 64,* 985-986.

Hoge's measure of intrinsic religious motivation and a death anxiety scale are completed by 103 white men age 61-88. The two measures are not correlated. Intrinsic religion may be a comfort to older men, but it does not appear to modify death anxiety. [2.2, 5.1]

SPIRITUALITY

<373> Birren, J. E. (1990). Spiritual maturity in psychological development. *Journal of Religious Gerontology, 7,* 41-53.

Observes that older men's importance has been displaced by technology in our informational society. Older men now would seem to have even more difficulty in seeking meaning in the later years of life, since our society contemplates whether the rib came from Eve. [2.3, 5.2]

<374> Carroll, L. P. , & Dyckman, K. M. (1986). *Chaos or creation: Spirituality in mid-life.* New York: Paulist Press.

Addresses how the religious and psychological trajectories may well follow a common developmental path. Contends that psychological developmental theory without the dimensions of faith is inadequate, and examines the experiences of mid-life and aging from a perspective which views the psychosocial reality as a "faith" reality. [1.5, 5.2]

<375> Clements, W. M. (1985-86). Aging and the dimensions of spiritual development. *Journal of Religion and Aging, 2,* 127-136.

Reviews how memory and prolepsis (the assumption of a future act or development as if it presently exists or has already been accomplished) contribute to elders' spiritual development. Proposes that the prevailing definition of time can inhibit spiritual development, but if the future is viewed as a series of discrete moments, then the creativity required for spiritual growth becomes possible. [5.2]

<376> Hateley, B. J. (1984). Spiritual well-being through life histories. *Journal of Religion and Aging, 1* (2), 63-71.

Explores the links between psychological well-being and spiritual well-being and describes a church adult education program in which life histories are used to enhance spiritual psychological well-being. The program appears particularly effective for those going through transitions such as career changes, divorce, or retirement, perhaps because it fosters reconciliation to the past, others, self, and God. [1.2, 5.2, 12.3]

<377> Jones, M. 1988. *Growing old--the ultimate freedom.* New York: Human Sciences Press.

Questioning the validity of many cultural stereotypes regarding the process of growing old, encourages the freedom to contemplate, to listen, to read, and to learn that is available to older men and women. Argues that these years provide an ideal opportunity for people to develop the capacity to think for themselves and to have the freedom to question much of the orthodoxy imposed by our current hierarchy of values. [5.2]

<378> Koenig, H. G., George, L. K., & Siegler, I. C. (1988). Use of religion and other emotion-regulating coping strategies among older adults. *The Gerontologist, 28,* 303-310.

Focusing on the use of religious behaviors for coping, investigates strategies used by older people in coping with stressful life changes. One hundred adults (involving equal numbers of men and women from the working class and upper middle class) age 55 to 80 in the Second Duke Longitudinal Study name the worst events of their whole lives, of the past 10 years, and at the present time, and tell how they had coped with these events. Overall, 289 stressful experiences are named, almost half of which are related to health. Religious coping behaviors are used most frequently, and nearly half the elders report that religious attitudes or actions help them cope. Private religious behaviors, such as trust and faith in God and prayer, are mentioned much more frequently than church-related or religious social activities. [2.2, 5.1, 5.2]

<379> Koenig, H. G., Cohen, J. J., Blazer, D. G., Pieper, C., & Meador, K. (1992). Religious coping and depression among elderly, hospitalized medically ill men. *American Journal of Psychiatry, 149*, 1693-1700.

Reports on the place of religious behavior and coping in lives of 850 hospitalized, medically ill older men. One out of five men reveal that religious thought and/or activity is the most important strategy they used to cope with illness, and depressive symptoms are inversely related to religious coping. In a six-month follow-up of 202 men, religious coping is the only baseline variable that predicts lower depression scores at follow-up. These findings demonstrate that religion has a buffering effect against adverse effects of environment stress and a positive effect on psychological stability. Associated with religious coping is being black, older, retired, having a religious affiliation, a high level of social support, and infrequent alcohol use. [2.2, 5.1, 5.2]

<380> Martin, D. S., & Fuller, W. G. (1991). Spirituality and aging: Activity key to "holiest" health care. *Activities, Adaptation and Aging, 15* (4), 37-50.

Residents in spiritual distress display the characteristics of helplessness, hopelessness, and withdrawal. Suggests that for elderly residents, faith is intertwined with the separate facets of religion and spirituality to keep them secured with symbol and ritual within the nursing home environment. "Holiest health care" fosters health-nurturing religion that keeps residents connected to their religious tradition. Clinebell's theory defines religion as having both left-brain functions (such as doing, works, seriousness, and loving God with one's mind) and right-brain functions (such as the experience of being, grace, playfulness, meditation, and communion); these can be applied in planning spiritual activities for residents. Describes the formation of a faith discussion group at a nursing home. [5.2, 12.3]

<381> McFadden, S. H. (1985). Attributes of religious maturity in aging people. *Journal of Religion and Aging, 1* (3), 39-48.

Examines the concept of religious maturity within the context of the life experience of aging people. Unlike descriptions which generally apply to healthy, active, middle-aged adults, the author's approach recognizes attributes of religious maturity in frail elderly persons as well. Reviewing and recreating the past through life reviews, the religiously mature aging person distinguishes between childhood religious objects and the experience of the transcendent in maturity. The older person becomes more open to the symbols, rituals, and myths of faith. By mourning losses in the present, the religiously mature older person has greater freedom to seek deeper spiritual awareness and a new understanding of time. [5.2]

<382> McSherry, E., Salisberg, S. R., Ciulla, M. R., & Tsuang, D. 1987. Spiritual resources in older hospitalized men. *Social Compass, 34,* **515-537.**

Examines how the spiritual resources of men ameliorated the adversity of hospitalization. Among the CABG (coronary artery bypass surgery; average age 62) patients, men self-rated as moderate to high in religiosity left the hospital earlier. Men's religious participation is characteristically low despite deep faith commitment. [5.2, 12.2]

<383> Moberg, D. O. (1990). Spiritual maturity and wholeness in the later years. *Journal of Religious Gerontology, 7,* **5-24.**

Although spirituality is very important to most older people, and although well-being and maturity are relevant to gerontological theories, consensus on the criteria for evaluating these three constructs is not yet complete. Mainstream gerontology largely ignores the issue and needs to integrate the importance of the spiritual into conceptions of elder's lives. [5.2]

<384> Payne, B. P. (1994). Faith development in older men. In E. Thompson (Ed.), *Older men's lives* **(pp. 85-103). Thousand Oaks, CA: Sage Publications.**

Draws on Erikson, Fowler, and Stokes to profile how men's faith practice and experience change and grow in late life. Theorizes that men shift the locus of their search for meaning in later life from external experiences toward inner ones. The providences of men's uneven faith development noticeably migrates from horizonal maturation (e.g., prochurch involvement) to vertical maturation (e.g., devotionalism, deep personal relationship with God). Theorizes that older men more likely decrease their behavioral (or horizonal) faithing and shift to more relational (or vertical) faithing when opportunities change, such as with retirement and caregiving for an ill wife. [1.5, 5.2]

<385> Rainbow, J. (1991). Spiritual and faith development in the later years. *Review and Expositor, 88,* **195-204.**

Examines the meaning of spirituality and quality aging from a pastoral perspective. Distinct from objective indicators of religiosity such as church attendance, spirituality is defined as, not one compartment of life, but the deepest dimension of all of life. [5.2]

<386> Shulik, R. A. (1988). Faith development in older adults. *Educational Gerontology, 14,* **291-301.**

Explains James Fowler's paradigm of faith development and applies it to a study of faith development in older adults. A sample of 20 men and 20 women age 60 and older finds little evidence to support the disengagement, life review, preparation for death, or philosophical development hypotheses of normal aging. Level of faith development is related to the degree to which the older person is aware of age-related changes and is also closely related to Kohlberg and Lovinger's measures of moral and ego development. Respondents who have achieved intermediate stages of faith development are less likely to be depressed than respondents whose developmental stages are either low or high. [1.5, 2.3, 5.2]

<387> Stokes, K. (1990). **Faith development in the adult life cycle.** *Journal of Religious Gerontology,* **7,** 167-184.

Interviews assessing over 1,000 adults' faith development throughout the adult life cycle are analyzed to test seven hypotheses. The results primarily demonstrate that faith development is not significantly related to age. Nor does it differ for men and women -- they are similar in the amount and nature of faith change, yet subtly different in the ways they experience faith. Men define faith as a set of beliefs and are more reserved in faith expression. Concludes that faith development trajectories for men and women become more similar in later life. [1.5, 5.2]

<388> Thibault, J. M., Ellor, J. W., & Netting, F. E. (1991). **Conceptual framework for assessing the spiritual functioning and fulfillment of older adults in long-term care settings.** *Journal of Religious Gerontology,* **7** (4), 29-45.

Spirituality refers to the manner in which a person integrates three domains --knowledge or belief system, inner life experiences, and exterior life and institutional activities in support of these beliefs. Service providers (N = 112) and 75 older adults age 61-89 are asked to identify those spiritual needs they would want nursing home staff to be aware of and what they would want to share with someone about their own lifelong spiritual journey. Results show great similarity between the responses of the professionals and those of the older adults in terms of their spiritual needs and the decision to share those needs. Having nursing home staff understand the importance of worship services and personal study resources for faith development is important. [5.2, 11.1]

<389> Weisman, C. B., & Schwartz, P. (1989). **Spirituality: An integral part of aging.** *Journal of Aging and Judaism,* **3** (3), 110-115.

Reviews the relationship between elders' spirituality and identity, and describes three models of Jewish spiritual expression -- behavioral, pietistic, and intellectual. Under the behavioral model, elders find structure and meaning by attending synagogue daily or by participating in other rituals and traditions. The pietistic model is expressed as a belief that God will take care, and this thought underlies an intense emotional bond and iden-tification with God. The intellectual model focuses on the fulfillment of spiritual yearnings as the elderly join rabbinical students in studying the Talmud. [5.2]

6

Stereotypes and Social Constructions

—◆—

AGEISM AND STEREOTYPING

<390> Baker, J. A., & Goggin, N. L. (1994). Portrayals of older adults in Modern
Maturity advertisements. *Educational Gerontology, 20* (2), 139-145.

Analyzes portrayals of older adults found in the full-page advertisements in Modern
Maturity from December 1987 to November 1991, and identifies stereotyping based on
age and gender. Finds 342 people depicted in 174 ads selected for analysis, but only
42% appear to be older adults. Nearly half of the people are men, and only 3% are
people of color. Latent content portrays old age as decreasing sexual attractiveness and
intimacy, older adults as dependent on children for love and purpose in life, and depicts
a predominance of products designed to minimize the effects of aging. [6.1]

<391> Bell, J. (1992). In search of a discourse on aging: The elderly on tele-
vision. *The Gerontologist, 32,* 305-311.

Analyzes the images of aging presented in five 1989 prime time television series which
have central elderly characters. Finds earlier stereotypes replaced by more positive
stereotypes portraying affluence, health, activeness, admiration, and sexiness. However, images still remain sexist. Men are far more likely to appear, and they are generally more active, powerful, and productive. Concludes that there are two universes
depicted -- a female universe of older women where there are no men, and a male universe where there are women, but no older women. [6.1]

<392> Braithwaite, V. A. (1986). Old age stereotypes: Reconciling contradic-
tions. *Journal of Gerontology, 41,* 353-360.

Tests the hypothesis that age stereotyping would occur when targets were disabled,
when information was minimal, and when the context was commonplace. Data are from
208 students on two judgment tasks. Finds both positive and negative age stereotyping
when the target was generalized (e.g., "the majority of old men") but not when it
provided specific information. Target's gender does not interact with age--elderly male
and female targets are perceived as equally more concerned with others and more
responsible than younger (age 25) counterparts, but less active and sociable. [6.1]

<393> **Brock, A. M., O'Neal, D. J., & Walker, M. L. (1978). Demythologizing the issues.** *Journal of Gerontological Nursing, 4* (6), 26-33.

In this discussion of stereotypes of aging, the ambiguity of men's aging and retirement are made clinically relevant. American society holds an ambiguous attitude toward retirement, which is viewed as a goal and reward by some, and by others is considered fraught with difficulties. It is deceptive to view retirement as a privilege. Misinformation about the sexual capacity of elderly men has also led to age-based stereotypes. This and other stereotypes create a situation in which old age is equated with social loss. [6.1, 6.2]

<394> **Brubaker, T. H., & Powers, E. A. (1976). The stereotype of old: A review and alternative approach.** *Journal of Gerontology, 31,* 441-447.

Observes that a negative stereotype of "old" has been emphasized, and how some researchers argue the negative stereotype is important for self-concept in late life. Questions the validity of this argument and presents a model more congruent with data. Analyzes forty-seven reports of research on stereotypes of old age, and finds that just 21 studies utilize older persons in the sample. Half of these are based on institutionalized or indigent aged. [6.1]

<395> **Bornstein, R. F. (1986). The number, identity, meaning, and salience of ascriptive attributes in adult person perception.** *International Journal of Aging and Human Development, 23,* 127-140.

Examines how many and which psychosocial attributes are utilized when someone engages in a comparison of stimulus persons. Data are from 211 men and 250 women (ages 20, 35, 50, 65, 80) comparing five adult-aged targets. Finds that regardless of the age or gender of the respondent group, only three target attributes are perceived as salient--age, gender, and autonomy. Very different salience is assigned to the three attributes and they are used in quite different ways to categorize the stimulus target. Perceived age is the most salient attribute, not gender. Perceived autonomy is also more salient than gender. [6.1, 6.2]

<396> **Dail, P. W. (1985). Prime time television portrayals of older adults in the context of family life.** *The Gerontologist, 28,* 700-706.

Investigates the portrayals of older adults in 12 family-oriented prime-time programs. Determines through content analysis 193 older adult characters' social interaction, emotional behavior, and cognitive, physical, and health status. Those older than age 55 are depicted more favorably than the middle-aged, and prime-time television reinforces the concept of later life being less difficult than the middle years. The findings also demonstrate men are much more favorably presented than women, revealing an image of men as stronger, more involved, . [6.1]

<397> **Elliott, J. (1984). The daytime television drama portrayal of older adults.** *The Gerontologist, 24,* 628-633.

Studies the representation of older adults in daytime serial dramas in 1979. Analyses reveal older adult actors comprise 8 percent of the characters, which is close to

population parameters. However, older men outnumber older women in serial char-
actors nearly two to one, and they are twice as likely to be married and cast as a
professional. Men engage in behaviors of looking and listening, problem solving, and
making statements, while women are nurturant or verbally aggressive. [6.1]

<398> Hummert, M. L. (1990). Multiple stereotypes of elderly and young adults:
     A comparison of structure and evaluations. *Psychology and Aging*, *5*, 182-
     193.

Examines how college students sort traits into groups when thinking about the age of an
adult. Analysis confirm the existence of distinct, multiple stereotypes of each age group.
Results also show attitudes varied with the stereotype activated; for example, older and
younger respondents exhibit more positive attitudes toward the positive categories.
[6.1]

<399> Hummert, M. L., Garstka, T. A., Shaner, J. L., & Strahm, S. (1994).
     Stereotypes of the elderly held by young, middle-aged, and elderly adults.
     Journal of Gerontology: Psychological Sciences, 49, P240-P249.

Extends research on multiple stereotypes of elders by examining the perceptions of
young, middle-age and elderly adults. Having 120 adults (age 18-85) generate lists of
traits on how they would describe the typical elderly adult, and another 120 sort the
listed traits into trait groupings, data show that older adults have more complex
representations of aging than do middle-age and younger adults. [6.1]

<400> Jackson, L. A., & Sullivan, L. A. (1988). Age stereotype disconfirming
     information and evaluations of old people. *Journal of Social Psychology*,
     128, 721-729.

Examines the age favorability bias among old respondents and the influence of a
target's gender on these ratings. Evaluations of three one-paragraph descriptions,
which are inconsistent with negative stereotypes about elder's social, physical and
psychological well-being are made by 102 elders and 81 young adults. When age
disconfirming information is present and does not confirm age stereotypes, respondents
more favorably rate the older targets. Only when targets are described as
psychologically competent are old men less favorably evaluated than old women, and
only by younger respondents. Age categorization, not gender, is more salient to the
younger participants. [6.1]

<401> Janelli, L. M. (1993). Grandparents' depictions in children's literature: A
     revisit. *Gerontology and Geriatrics Education, 14* (2), 43-52.

Reviews 37 children's storybooks copyrighted 1985-1990 and determines what changes
have occurred in the depictions of grandparents since the earlier, 1988 review of 73
books copyrighted 1966-1984. Found in the previous review that grandfathers appear
more individual than grandmothers, yet grandmothers and grandfathers are depicted
stereotypically. Content analysis of the 22 books on grandmothers and 15 on grandfathers reveals that grandparent characters still are depicted in stereotypic terms. The
grandfather characters are balding, have gray hair, and wear glasses; they are likely to

be involved in teaching activities, while the grandmothers are more likely to be cooking and providing affection to grandchildren. Only one book focuses on a black grandfather. The author cautions that educators need to be aware that attitudes toward the elderly and aging develop early and, once formed, influence thoughts and behavior in adulthood. [6.1, 8.3]

<402> Kite, M. E., & Johnson, B. T. (1988). **Attitudes toward older and younger adults: A meta-analysis.** *Psychology and Aging, 3,* 233-244.

Conducts a meta-analysis of the literature on attitudes toward elders to examine if the elderly are viewed more negatively than younger persons. Demonstrates that attitudes toward elders are more negative. But smaller differences are found when personality traits are compared and specific information is provided about the target person. These findings suggest age is less important in determining attitudes toward elders than other types of information. [6.1]

<403> Kite, M. E., Deaux, K., & Miele, M. (1991). **Stereotypes of young and old: Does age outweigh gender.** *Psychology and Aging, 6,* 19-27.

Comments how few studies examine directly the interaction of age and gender stereotyping. Determines stereotypes of age and gender using 35- and 65-year-old men and women as target persons. Finds the age stereotypes are more pronounced than gender stereotypes, particularly when attributes are freely generated by respondents. Older men are distinguished more from younger men and younger people, less from older women. Together, older men and women are judged less likely to possess masculine characteristics, whereas judgments about feminine characteristics are largely unaffected by the target's age. Some gender stereotyping is evident: All men are thought to possess masculine traits, role behaviors, and physical characteristics, whereas women possess feminine. No double standard of aging is observed. [6.1]

<404> Kogan, N., & Mills, M. (1992). **Gender influences on age cognitions and preferences: Sociocultural or sociobiological?.** *Psychology and Aging, 7,* 98-106.

Observes that the study of attitudes toward aging and elders is now four decades old, but understudied is the role of gender. Reviews the available research addressing gender effects on age cognitions and evaluations. Sontag's double standard of aging--proposing more negative consequences of aging in women in contrast to men--serves as a point of departure. Research using attitude-scale, semantic differential, and person-perception methodologies points to sex-of-target, sex-of-subject, and target-subject interaction effects. Findings are not completely consistent, but the evidence suggests that age is a more salient dimension for men's evaluations and cognitions than for women. Men exhibit a stronger youth bias. Discusses the consistent of the findings with an evolutionary hypothesis, and urges research which focuses on proximal determinants. [6.1, 9.1]

<405> Lachman, M. E., & McArthur, L. Z. (1986). **Adulthood age differences in causal attributions for cognitive, physical, and social performance.** *Psychology and Aging, 1,* 127-132.

Poor performance and failures by an elder are generally attributed to internal and stable factors such as inability, whereas poor performance by the young is attributed to external and unstable factors such as bad luck. Investigates 42 young and 39 elderly men's and women's causal attributions for their own and for another person's hypothetical performance in three realms--cognitive, physical, and social. The pattern of results give an unflattering view of the elderly. However, when attributions for good v. poor performance by elders are compared, elders are credited for good performances as equally as they are blamed for poor performances. [6.1, 9.1]

<406> Larson, G. W., Hayslip, B. Jr., & Wright-Thomas, K. (1992). **Changes in voice onset time in young and older men.** *Educational Gerontology, 18,* 285-297.

Listener perception of age in voice and subsequent judgment of speaker characteristics contribute to the social constructions of age. Investigates the effect of age on the articulatory-laryngeal adjustments required for speech, and finds a clear age-related effect on speech, with older men readily distinguished. These findings demonstrate that acoustics can distinguish groups of younger from older male speakers. Voice characteristics may prove to be a major factor influencing listener perception. [2.1, 6.1, 6.2]

<407> Milligan, W. L., Prescott, L., Powell, D. A., & Furchtgott, E. (1989). **Attitudes towards aging and physical health.** *Experimental Aging Research, 15,* 33-41.

Examines whether a component of negative attitudes toward the aged is related to the greater occurrence of physical illness in elders. Vignettes of four individuals who differ in age and physical health are presented to people who differ in age and gender. Each participant reads one profile and rates the target on a semantic differential scale of attitudes towards aging. No participant gender effects are found. All three age groups-- young (29 or younger), middle-aged (30-49), and older (50 years and older) rate the two age-targets in poor health more negatively than healthy target persons. Further, more negative attitudes toward the aged are likely to occur in older than younger respondents regardless of health status. [2.1, 6.1]

<408> Minnigerode, F. A., & Lee, J. A. (1978). **Young adults' perceptions of social sex roles across the life span.** *Sex Roles, 4,* 563-569.

Gender roles are seldom examined from a life-span perspective which includes middle and later adulthood. The present study examines how 50 male and 50 female undergraduates perceive gender at five target ages across the life span. Ten age-sex targets are rated on semantic differential scales assessing potency, activity, and evaluative dimensions. During early and middle adulthood gender differences are attributable to potency, or masculinity-femininity. In later life gender roles are judged to be more similar than at any other point in the life span. [6.1]

<409> Mundorf, N., & Brownell, W. (1990).   Media preferences of older and younger adults. *The Gerontologist, 30,* 685-691.

Updates research on television viewing and magazine reading of older adults, and compares it with media preferences of college students. Older adults (N = 74; mean age = 72) report higher levels of television viewing than college students (N = 149). Both age groups show preferences to television characters their own age. Gender preferences are less clear-cut. Men and older adults prefer members of their own gender and the programs featuring them. Entertainment is the primary motive for television viewing, however more men report watching television for information, men report markedly less daytime viewing, and men use the television less for companionship. These patterns suggest older adults are not a homogenized viewing population and are more similar to those of younger adults than results of previous research would have predicted. [6.1]

<410> Parr, W. V., & Seigert, R. (1993).   Adults' conceptions of everyday memory failures in others: Factors that mediate the effects of target age. *Psychology and Aging, 8,* 599-605.

Investigates 100 younger and 100 older adults' conceptions of memory failures in targets age 20, 40, 60, and 80. Participates rate how likely the memory failures are a lack of effort or lack of ability. Finds the double-standard of memory-failure appraisal. There is a decrease in lack-of-effort ratings and an increase in lack-of-ability ratings with targets' increasing age. This double-standard is more a continuum, beginning as young as 40, rather than a simple prejudice against elders. Target age is more salient for older participants, and equally salient for men and women. Both men and women evaluate opposite sex targets more harshly and their own gender more favorably, rating memory failures in same sex targets as less likely a result of lack of ability. [6.1]

<411> Revenson, T. A. (1989).   Compassionate stereotyping of elder patients by physicians: Revising the social contact hypothesis. *Psychology and Aging, 4,* 230-234.

Examines age stereotyping by physicians and whether amount of contact with elder patients affects stereotyping. Rheumatologists evaluate a 53 or an 83-year-old target patient on a number of dimensions including psychological adjustment and need for support and information. Targets' age and physicians' degree of contact with elderly patients have few direct effects, but their interaction yields a strong and consistent finding: The elderly patient is rated as less adjusted, autonomous, and instrumental and in greater need of support and information by high-contact physicians. Findings are explained by the reverse social contact hypothesis. Only a female target was rated, thus gender differences in the prevalence of specific illness in later life may determine response more than age. [6.1, 12.2]

<412> Schmidt, D. F., & Boland, S. M. (1986).   Structure of perceptions of older adults: Evidence of multiple stereotypes. *Psychology and Aging, 1,* 255-260.

Determines we hold complex (or multiple) stereotypes of the elderly. Subjects are college students. In the first phase of the study, stereotype content is sampled by asking students to describe the typical old person. In the next phase, other students sort the traits identified into one or more groups of similarly defined older adults. The tree diagrams of trait clusters reveal positive traits for elders are stereotypically masculine (e.g., tough, distinguished, sage) and negative traits are feminine (e.g., bag lady, dependent). [6.1]

<413> Sherman, S. R. (1985). Sex role stereotypes of middle and old age. *Journal of Social Service Research*, 8, 23-35.

Prior research on gender role stereotypes makes little reference to age of targets. Examines 534 university students assessments of targets of different ages and sex -- a middle-aged or old man, woman, or person -- on measures of stereotyping. Findings do not suggest many gender stereotypes. A gender difference for the target rated is found on only three adjective pairs, and age-sex interactions are found on three. [6.1]

<414> Silverman, M. (1977). The old man as woman: Detecting stereotypes of aged men with a femininity scale. *Perceptual and Motor Skills*, 44, 336-338.

There are some indications that interests and attitudes of men become more feminine with age. In this study, college students rate women in general and older men significantly higher in femininity than men at four younger ages. Findings affirm that women in general and older men are viewed through the same "femininity" stereotype, and perceived femininity increases in men as a function of age. [6.1]

<415> Turner, B. F., & Turner, C. B. (1991). Bem sex-role inventory stereotypes for men and women varying in age and race among National Register psychologists. *Psychological Reports*, 69, 931-944.

Explores gender stereotypes for men and women who differ in age and race. Psychologists (N = 554) rate a mature, health, socially competent individual in one of 18 target groups--a black or race-unspecified man, women, or adult in their late 20s, 40s, 60s. Old targets are viewed as less agentic, male targets are rated as less feminine and more masculine. Older men are perceived as more agentic than like-aged women among presumably-white targets, but not among black targets, and old presumably-white men are viewed as no less self-governing than middle-age targets. [6.1]

<416> Vernon, J. A., Williams, J. A. Jr., Phillips, T., & Wilson, J. (1990). Media stereotyping: A comparison of the way elderly women and men are portrayed on prime-time television. *Journal of Women and Aging*, 2, 55-68.

Investigates the ways elderly women and men are portrayed on prime-time television. Content analysis of 139 prime-time programs during one week in the fall of 1987 and again in the summer of 1988, reveal that older adults, particularly older women, are underrepresented in commercial television. There is a preponderance of the older, middle-aged man in leading television roles and a relative lack of appearance of middle-aged women in such roles. When portrayed, older adults most often are depicted in negative, stereotypical ways, but the presentations are not as marked a distortion as has been previously reported. Negative images are being replaced by more positive images. [6.1]

<417> Walsh, R. P., & Connor, C. L. (1979). Old men and young women: How objectively are their skills assessed? *Journal of Gerontology, 34*, 561-568.

Research on societal expectations for men to be more competent than women and to perform well suggest that expectations vary by age as much as gender. In this study, 74 undergraduates (37 men) evaluate an essay describing a work of art attributed to a 25 year-old male or female, or a 64 year-old male or female. The interaction of the target's age and gender is significant. Young women and older men are targets of subtle prejudices which cause their work to be assessed unobjectively. The implications seem particularly important for older men since retirement is now based on when the person is no longer able to perform effectively. [6.1]

SOCIAL CONSTRUCTIONS OF AGING

<418> Chinen, A. B. (1987). Fairy tales and psychological development in late life: A cross-cultural hermeneutic study. *The Gerontologist, 27*, 340-346.

Discusses how a distinct minority of fairy tales feature older adults, and analyzes their recurrent themes. Of 2,500 fairy tales located in cross-cultural collections and reviewed, just 2 percent feature older adults. They can be called elder tales because they show what this stage of development ideally entails -- more complex judgments and responsibility for one's own shortcomings. Discusses six themes arising from elder tales (e.g., poverty, transcendence, worldly wisdom), and concludes that elder tales speak to both the child and grandparent, unifying magic and wisdom in later life. [6.2]

<419> Covey, H. C. (1988) Historical terminology used to represent older people. *The Gerontologist, 28*, 291-297.

Traces semantically the words people use to represent older people, aging, and the effects of aging by using the Oxford English Dictionary and other sources. Gender is a critical factor in the selection of terminology for the old. The English language has a long history of separating old men from old women, and terms for old men address stereotypes such as being conservative, feeble, stingy, incompetent, narrow-minded. Common descriptors in the 16th century included baldhead and gaffer. Terms sometimes connote the positive tone of being wise and respected. Generally, terms are a reflection of how older men were viewed, and the pattern across time is a decline in status and increased focus on the debilitative effects of aging. [6.2]

<420> Covey, H. C. (1989). Old age portrayed by the ages-of-life models from the Middle Ages to the 16th century. *The Gerontologist, 29*, 692-698.

Examines the ages of life portrayed in the literature and the arts of the late Middle ages and Renaissance to assess how aging and old age were routinely perceived in earlier times. Most ages-of-life models have elements of both continuity and abrupt change, of ambiguity and inconsistency. Most models are traced to earlier Greek explanations of the life span, and surprising consistency of what is defined as age appropriate behavior exists, with old age a time of contemplation, spiritual restoration, poor health, and miserliness. Most ages-of-life models are masculine constructions. [6.2]

<421> Fiedler, L. A. (1979). Eros and Thanatos: Old age in love. In D. D. Van Tassel (Ed.), *Aging, death, and the completion of being* (pp. 235-254). Philadelphia: University of Pennsylvania Press.

Myths of old men in love are explored through examples from literature, films, drama, and song. The plight of mythic old men in love represents the tension between Eros and Thanatos (carnal love and physical death) which determines the basic rhythms of human life. This depiction reveals the central absurdity of being human, of a desire that cannot be denied without denying the fragility of the flesh upon which satisfaction of that desire depends. Examples are presented from Shakespeare, who often addressed the problem of the aged in love with youth. [6.2]

<422> Kastenbaum, R. (1989). Old men created by young artists: Time-transcendence in Tennyson and Picasso. *International Journal of Aging and Human Development, 28,* 81-104.

Observes how Tennyson and Picasso created in their youth masterpieces that envisioned old men. Explores the context within which these early masterpieces were created, the style and substance of the works themselves, and the possible relationships between the artists' young and old selves. Although Tennyson and Picasso are "exceptional cases," many other people also transcend their momentary position on the lifespan and, by acts of empathic imagination, "commune" with past and future selves. Developmental theory might enrich itself by considering these processes and their functions and consequences. [1.5, 6.2]

<423> Kastenbaum, R. (1990). The age of saints and the saintliness of age. *International Journal of Aging and Human Development, 30,* 95-118.

Examines the longevity among saints and includes a discussion of the saint as a possible model for the old person. Uses a sample of 487 saints (369 males) drawn from reference sources to reveal an interaction between gender and historical period. Martyrdom is twice as common among the males, who are likely to be put to death in their forties, rather than dying young as are female martyrs. Male saints have a mean longevity of 69.9 years--literally the proverbial "three score and ten." Saints, especially the men, have a longevity advantage throughout most of history. A trend is also noted for the age of male saints--the number of very old saints has diminished, and centenarians have been absent for more than seven hundred years. [6.2]

<424> Kebric, R. B. (1988). Old age, the ancient military, and Alexander's army: Positive examples for a graying America. *The Gerontologist, 28,* 298-302.

Introduces the false belief that few people in antiquity lived to old age, then reviews evidence that elders formed a sizable segment of the community and were productive, active citizens. Examples from ancient Greece and Rome, where the working aged were common, make clear that physically fit elders who wished to remain active continued to do so, as in their participation in the military and battle. Only the wealthy could consider retiring. Apparently, age was less visible than gender. [6.2]

<425> Montepare, J. M., & Lachman, M. E. (1989). "You're only as old as you feel": Self-perceptions of age, fears of aging, and life satisfaction from adolescence to old age. *Psychology and Aging, 4,* 73-78.

Identifying developmental patterns in age identities would help clarify whether older adults' age perceptions reflect stable self-views or changes in self-perceptions. Examines subjective age identification from adolescence to old age, and fears about one's own aging in 188 people ages 14 to 83. Respondents judge how old they felt, look, act, and desire to be. Teens hold older subjective age identities, whereas middle-age and older adults reported young age identities. Men report older age identities than women across the adult years. No strong relation is observed between older men's subjective age and their present life satisfaction. [1.1, 6.2]

<426> Nelson, E. A., & Dannefer, D. (1992). Aged heterogeneity: Fact or fiction? The face of diversity in gerontological research. *The Gerontologist, 32,* 17-23.

Gerontological research examining age-related changes in individuals' lives typically reports outcomes which ignore the importance of the increasing variability in the elderly population. Examines the degree of attention given in 185 journal articles published from 1982 to 1987 to individual differences, and reports that two-thirds of the studies did indicate a pattern of increasing variability with age. However, the effect of gender and gender-by-age interactions are not discussed in the review. [6.2]

<427> Troll, L. E. (1988). New thoughts on old families. *The Gerontologist, 28,* 586-591.

Uses autobiographic information to illustrate how generational and gender positions influence someone's perspective on family organization and family relations. Raises four questions about gender in later life which remain uncharted theoretically and empirically. For example, a gender-sensitive (and feminist) perspective envisions self only as the child in family life, not as a competent old parent, a sibling, a grandparent. Gerontologists study old women only from this single frame, and rarely independent of a comparison to old men. Introduces an "omega" view of family systems and older mothers as subjects rather than an "object," and provides a new perspective on thinking about age and gender in families. By illustration, urges the study of older men as subjects rather than comparative objects. [1.5, 6.2]

7

Relationships and Social Life

— ♦ —

SOCIAL PARTICIPATION

<428> Albert, S. M., & Moss, M. (1990). Consensus and the domain of personal relations among older adults. *Journal of Social and Personal Relationships, 7, 353-369.*

Older men and women (N = 225) rate a set of personal relations attributes according to their own interaction with friends and relatives. Correlates each individual's profile with every other in order to determine how similar older men and women are. This strategy provides a measure of consensus in thinking about personal relationships. Although the degree of consensus does not differ significantly across gender or marital groups, mental health correlates show men more disadvantaged, providing partial support for gender-specific interpersonal cultures. [7.1, 7.3]

<429> Hammond, R. J., & Muller, G. O. (1992). The late-life divorced: Another look. *Journal of Divorce and Remarriage, 17,* 135-150.

Determines the prevalence rates of divorce among the 397 elderly men and 936 women and investigates the effects of marital dissolution in late life. The research uses data from the National Survey of Families and Households. Principally finds that older men are less likely to turn to others for emotional support during separation than are younger men or older women, and formerly married men report less happiness and poorer adjustment scores. [1.4, 7.1]

<430> Herzog, A. R., & Morgan, J. N. (1992). Age and gender differences in the value of productive activities. *Research on Aging, 14,* 169-198.

Expands the definition of productivity beyond paid labor to include many forms of unpaid work (such as housework, formal volunteer work, informal help of relatives and friends). Estimates empirically elders' complete productivity, and determines the extent to which many activities often performed without pay are actually productive. Finds older men and women report at least as many hours and contribute in major ways to the nation's productivity. Gender differences in the value of work indicate that men earn actual wages and hourly dollar values three times greater than women, yet the gender difference converges with aging. [7.1, 10.2]

<431> McGuire, F. A.   (1982).   Leisure time, activities, and meanings: A comparison of men and women in late life. In N. J. Osgood (Ed.), *Life after work: Retirement, leisure, recreation, and the elderly*. New York: Praeger Publishers.

Reviews the available literature on gender differences in older adults' perceptions of the amount of leisure time they have, types of leisure activities pursued, and the meaning of leisure. Men have more leisure time than women throughout life, and this difference carries over beyond retirement. Leisure activity patterns of older men differ markedly from women's, but the differences are due primarily to gender and not age. Despite differences in the activity involvement of men and women, the meaning attached to leisure is highly individualized and more dependent on personality than on age, gender, or social class. [7.1]

<432> Peterson, S. A., & Somit, A. (1992). The political behavior of older American blacks. *The Gerontologist, 32*, 592-600.

Evaluates three competing explanations for the political behavior of black Americans age 55 and older in a subsample of the 1987 General Social Survey (N = 157). Finds older men have greater political interest than older women, and older African-Americans' political interest is directly related to level of participation. The socioeconomic (isolation) model is a better predictor of older African-American political interest, activity, and alienation than the ethnic community and empowerment theories. [7.1]

<433> Pohjolainen, P. (1991). Social participation and life-style: A longitudinal and cohort study. *Journal of Cross Cultural Gerontology, 6*, 109-117.

Examines the relationship of socioeconomic status and health to social participation, describing the changes occurring in social participation during the retirement years for cohorts born in 1905-06, 1909-10, 1917-18, and 1921-22. While social membership remains basically unchanged, formal social participation declines with age among both men and women. There are no cohort differences for men's formal social participation, whereas for women social participation is higher in the younger cohorts. [7.1]

<434> Webb, L., Delany, J. J., & Young, L. R. (1989). Age, interpersonal attraction, and social interaction: A review and assessment. *Research on Aging, 11*, 107-123.

Reviews more than 40 research reports on attraction and aging. Concludes that elders prefer to routinely associate with middle-age and older adults more than younger adults, regardless of the physical attractiveness of the target person, and marital satisfaction appears related to the perceive attractiveness of the husband, not wife. [7.1]

VOLUNTEERING

<435> Fischer, K., Rapkin, B. D., & Rappaport, J. (1991). Gender and work

history in the placement and perceptions of elder community volun.
Psychology of Women Quarterly, 15, 261-279.

Explores how 169 elder volunteers (39 men) from different career paths interpret the leadership and nonleadership volunteer jobs. An interaction effect between gender and type of volunteer job is noted. When men are leaders, their sense of interpersonal feedback is higher than when they are nonleaders, but their sense of influence and autonomy is lower. Women in leadership jobs fell more influential and autonomous than their peers in nonleadership jobs. Work history is a significant predictor of leadership jobs for men, but not for women. Men with prestigious preretirement work histories perceive their volunteer roles as less influential than men who have been in lower status jobs before retirement. [7.2, 10.2]

<436> Fischer, L. R., Mueller, D. P., & Cooper, P. W. (1991). Older volunteers: A discussion of the Minnesota Senior Study. *The Gerontologist, 31,* 183-194.

The known effect of gender on volunteering is mixed. Some studies report men volunteer less; some show no gender difference in likelihood of volunteering, even though men spend somewhat fewer hours volunteering; still other studies show the greatest numbers of volunteers are from men who do somewhat different types of volunteer work. In an original study, more than half (52%) of older Minnesotans volunteer, which is considerably higher than is been found in national surveys. Older men and women are about equally likely to be volunteers, however they tend to differ in the specific types of helping they choose to do. These differences largely conform to gender expectations -- older men doing "downstairs/outside" work more commonly than visiting or providing person-to-person care. Men are somewhat more likely to work for citizenship-type organizations than churches or social welfare and health organizations, and they spend many fewer hours per month volunteering (5 v. 15) than women. [7.2]

<437> Okun, M. A. (1993). Predictors of volunteer status in a retirement community. *International Journal of Aging and Human Development, 36,* 57-74.

Contributing to the research on predictors of elders' volunteering, this study uses discriminant analysis to identify three types of volunteers. Actual volunteers are equally likely to be men as women, attend church frequently, be free of activity limitations due to health, have volunteered previously, and belong to several clubs and organizations. By comparison, latent volunteers engage in informal religious behavior, attend church about once a month, are very satisfied with their neighborhood, and are younger (about age 70) than other elder volunteers. Conditional volunteers engage infrequently in informal religious behavior, are also very satisfied with their neighborhood, and have no activity limitations due to health. [5.1, 7.2]

<438> Patterson, S. L. (1987). Older rural natural helpers: Gender and site differences in the helping process. *The Gerontologist, 27,* 639-644.

Investigates the characteristics of 80 older rural "natural helper" caregivers. Although the men (N = 38) are similar on demographic variables to the women, there are marked gender differences in helper motivation. Older men reveal a moral obligatory approach to helping and women show the caring, nurturing approach. Men also appear to use a narrower repertoire of helping styles and face a narrower variety of problems. Their "natural" helping style offers friends and neighbors a unique gender style which is based on their separateness and ethic of protecting the rights of others. [7.2]

FRIENDSHIPS

<439> Adams, R. G. (1994). In E. Thompson (Ed.), *Older men's lives* **(pp. 159-177). Thousand Oaks, CA: Sage Publications.**

Proposes that to understand older men's friendships, it is necessary to study the effects of gender among older adults, as well as the interactive effects of age and gender across the life course. Using a new integrative framework, reviews what can be gleaned from 28 friendship research studies which include a subsample of older men. Patterns of older men have greater gender heterogeneity in their friendship networks compared to older women, and are less likely to confide in friends. As men age, they maintain friendships longer. Concludes by reviewing directions further work could undertake methodologically and conceptually. [7.3]

<440> Connidis, I. A., & Davis, L. (1990). Confidants and companions in later life: The place of family and friends. *Journals of Gerontology: Social Sciences,* **45, S141-S149.**

Determines the relative importance of friends and various family members (spouse, children, siblings) as confidants and as companions in a sample of 400 older persons. Unlike prior studies, finds children make up a larger proportion of the confidant network of men than of women (43 vs. 35 percent). Spouses and friends are the next most important confidants for men, although not quite one-fifth report they confide in friends or spouses. The companion network is composed of markedly different people. Half of the men identify the spouse as a companion, followed by friends. Distinguishing types of networks reveals spouses are in men's companion rather than confidant network. [7.3, 7.5, 8.4]

<441> Fischer, C. S., & Oliker, S. J. (1983). A research note on friendship, gender, and the life cycle. *Social Forces,* **62, 124-133.**

Prior research increasingly suggests that the personal relations of men and women differ. Investigates the prevalence and types of friendships for 1,050 adults (over age 18), probing for gender differences in the friendship patterns. Finds the differences are contingent on stage in the life cycle. This interaction effect is evidence for a structural and a dispositional explanation of the gender differences. The data reveal few global gender differences in personal relations (men are more involved with coworkers and women with relatives) yet numerous differences in different phases of life cycle. During early marriage and parenthood, women's friendships diminished relative to men's. In the postparental years, men's friendships diminished relative to women's. [1.4, 7.3]

<442> Fox, M., Gibbs, M., & Auerbach, D. (1985). Age and gender dimensions of friendship. *Psychology of Women Quarterly,* **9, 489-501.**

Depth interviewing of samples of 5 men and 5 women at three ages--age 65-75, 35-55, and 18-22--finds men and women of different ages describe friendship in superficially similar ways. Beneath the surface similarities, however, gender reveals men at all ages are less expressive in their friendships, with low levels of empathy and altruism. Within-gender differences across age also appear. Men develop greater concern and thoughtfulness in friendship with greater age, and women show more tolerance and less confrontation of their friends with greater age. [7.3]

<443> Hatch, L. R., & Bulcroft, K. A. (1992). Contact with friends in later life: Disentangling the effects of gender and marital status. *Journal of Marriage and the Family, 54,* 222-232.

Compares groups of widowed, divorced or separated, and never-married men and women age 60-65 in the Retirement History Study on three dimensions of friendship contacts. Men have larger friendship networks--seeing or talking with a larger number of friends, yet men have less frequent contact with friends than women. The combined effects of gender and marital status are more revealing than direct effects of gender or marital status separately. Divorced or separated men have more friends than widowers or never married, yet widowers have more frequent contact. Frequency of friendship contact declines with age in all three marital groups. [7.3]

<444> Johnson, C. L., & Troll, L. E. (1994). Constraints and facilitators of friendships in late late life. *The Gerontologist, 34,* 79-87.

Analyzes friendship patterns of individuals age 85 and older (77% women). Despite high levels of disability and loss of age peers, the majority of elders are in frequent contact with friends and have a close friend. Increasing disability over the 31 months replaces gender and morale as predictors of friendship activity. The gender differences found in most friendship data at young ages are absent when disability increases. Apparently the differences in life style between younger men and women that contribute to differences in friendship are less apparent in the life styles of the oldest old. [7.3]

<445> Jones, D. C., & Vaughan, K. (1990). Close friendships among senior adults. *Psychology and Aging, 5,* 451-457.

Evaluates the relative contributions of personal, affective, and social exchange characteristics to satisfaction with best friend among 76 elders (23 married men, 24 married women, 29 single women). The older men (and the married women) identify, on average, 7 friends and a best friend of 21 years. Closeness ratings of best friends are equally strong for the older married men and women. Behaviorally, two-thirds of these men contact their best friend on a weekly basis, compared to 90% of the older married women and 80% of the single women. Communal orientation enhances satisfaction, but exchange orientation is not related to friendship satisfaction. [7.3]

<446> Mullins, L. C., & Mushel, M. (1992). The existence and emotional closeness of relationships with children, friends, and spouses: The effect of loneliness among older persons. *Research on Aging, 14,* 448-470.

Hypothesizes that the emotional commitment to the relationships older persons have with their children, their friends, and their spouses is related to their loneliness. Finds the loneliness varies with gender, health status, and economic condition, but not age.

Previous research indicates men are either less lonely than women or there was no difference. The greater loneliness among men in this study is explained by their reticent in expressing needs and a relocation effect. Elders recent migration to Florida may provide social integration without emotional support. The lack of influence by children and spouses on emotional loneliness also raises the question of whether kin are as important as friends in reducing the loneliness of emotional isolation. [2.3, 7.3]

<447> O'Connor, P. (1993). Same-gender and cross-gender friendships among the frail elderly. *The Gerontologist, 33,* 24-30.

Observes that platonic cross-gender friendships are not the exclusive prerogative of widows. The majority of frail elders' friends are peers in age and thus are not romantic or "charity" relationships. Same-gender friendships are more likely to occur among the non-househound. They are social, identity enhancing, and rooted in shared activities and past memories. [7.3]

<448> Powers, E. A., & Bultena, G. L. (1976). Sex differences in intimate friendships of old age. *Journal of Marriage and the Family, 38,* 739-747.

In a sample of 234 adults age 70 and older, assess the nature and prominence of intimate friendships in the social world of older men and women. Six factors which are potentially important for the intimate friendship patterns are examined: marital status, education, employment status, socioeconomic level, health, and social involvement. Contrary to stereotypes, men have more frequent social contacts than women, but a smaller proportion of their interaction is with intimate friends. There is little gender differentiation in the characteristics of intimate friendships in late life, although it is suggested that the motivation for formation and maintenance of intimate ties may differ for aged men and women. [7.3]

<449> Reisman, J. M. (1988). An indirect measure of the value of friendship for aging men. *Journals of Gerontology: Psychological Sciences, 43,* P109-P110.

Assesses the value of friendship for a group of aging men who are college graduates from the Harvard class of 1930. Analysis of the content of the autobiographical sketches published in the 25th and 50th anniversary reports of the graduating class indicates that married men mention (or value) friendship significantly less than career or family. There is evidence of an increase in casual friendly relations with more leisure time in old age, but no indication of an increase in close friendships. [7.3]

<450> Roberto, K. A., & Kimboko, P. J. (1988). Friendships in later life: Definitions and maintenance patterns. *International Journal of Aging and Human Development, 28,* 9-19.

Examines the meaning and maintenance of friend relationships in later life for men (N = 41) and women (N = 74) age 60 and older. While older men and women tend to agree on the characteristics of a friend, they have distinct perceptions of their current involvement with friends, they seem to different in the underlying subjective frameworks used to define another person as a friend, and gender differences emerge when they are asked to differentiate between a "friend" and a "close friend." Older men are less likely to consider friends made earlier in their lives as still part of their friend network, and they are less likely to focus on the relationship that is shared, but instead focused on the psychological qualities of the other person or the social similarities shared. It is likely that men, especially if married, have little need to go outside the family for closeness or help. [7.3]

<451> Roberto, K. A., & Scott, J. P. (1986). Friendships of older men and women: Exchange patterns and satisfaction. *Psychology and Aging, 1*, 103-109.

Examines the relation between perceived equity of exchanges and friendship satisfaction in a sample of 110 older men and women. Respondents discuss their best friend and one other friend. Men are involved in more equitable relationships with best and other friends than women. For men and women, perceived equity is a significant predictor of friendship satisfaction in the case of the other friend only. Overbenefited men in best-friendships express the greater amount of satisfaction. Because equity theory does not predict gender differences, the authors hypothesize men's less "depth-based" friendships, which emphasize shared activities and interests, set the stage for different equity considerations. [7.3]

DATING AND REMARRIAGE

<452> Bulcroft, K. A., & O'Connor, M. (1986). The importance of dating relationships on quality of life for older persons. *Family Relations, 35*, 397-401.

Interviews persons age 60 and older who are currently dating, and finds the dating relationship is a very significant one. It is the companionate more than passionate nature of the relationships which is important. The dating role does not replace formal spousal roles, nor does it duplicate roles within social networks. Older men stress the importance of dating as a means for intimacy need fulfillment and self disclosure rather than an opportunity to enhance prestige among peers. [7.4]

<453> Bulcroft, K. A., Bulcroft, R. A., Hatch, L. R., & Borgatta, E. F. (1989). Antecedents and consequences of remarriage in later life. *Research on Aging, 11*, 82-106.

Reviews the often made proposal that marriage serves to buffer stress, provide social support, and favorably affect well-being. Examines possible explanations for why older men themselves remarry using data from the Retirement History Study. Finds just two predictors--the fewer the number of people in the older man's household and shorter the length of time widowed/divorced are both related to remarriage rates. More recently singled men who live alone are more likely to remarry. Subjective health also seems to be positively related; men in better health remarry. After remarriage, however, health and happiness improve less for the husbands and more for their wives. [2.3, 2.4, 7.4]

<454> Bulcroft, R. A., & Bulcroft, K. A. (1991). The nature and functions of dating in later life. *Research on Aging, 13*, 244-260.

Argues that dating in the later stages of the life course has been ignored by researchers, but is taken seriously by older adults. Identifies factors that are predictors of dating for elders and whether dating affects psychological well-being using data from the National Survey of Families and Households. The strongest predictor is gender, with men significantly more likely to engage in dating. Organizational participation (but not work involvement or religious participation) increased men's likelihood of dating, and there is some suggestion that dating may be more emotionally rewarding for men. [7.4]

<455> McElhaney, L. J. (1992). Dating and courtship in the later years: A neglected topic of research. *Generations, 17,* 21-23.

Provides an overview of the sparse, available research on dating and courtship in later life. Perhaps 30 percent of previously married older men and 7 percent of the women report one date in the previous month. New relationships in later life are more likely to involve specific expectations for partners and to place more emphasis on companionship and less on sexuality. Reasons for dating reported by older people include selection of a marital partner and maintenance of social activity. Dating may be a realistic option only for older men, given the imbalance in the sex ratio. [7.4]

<456> Vinick, B. H. (1978). Remarriage in old age. *Family Coordinator, 27,* 359-363.

Examines what influences the remarriage among 24 couples who range in age from 60 to 84 years. Older men are more traumatized by the loss of spouse than older women, due to their prior lower degree of family and friend involvement, their simultaneous loss of work and spouse, and their inexperience in housekeeping roles. Not unexpectedly, more men report they feel lonely during widowhood. Remarried couples are most often introduced by a mutual acquaintance -- that is, the socially active are more likely to remarry. Companionship is the strongest motivation inducing people to remarry, and for men, health and morale affect marriage satisfaction. Most remarried couples report satisfaction with the new marriage. [7.4, 8.4]

SOCIAL NETWORKS AND SUPPORT

<457> Antonucci, T. C., & Akiyama, H. (1987). An examination of sex differences in social support among older men and women. *Sex Roles, 17,* 737-749.

Examines differences in married men's and women's qualitative and quantitative social support and its effects on well-being. Data are from 214 men and 166 women age 50-95 who participated in the Supports for the Elderly Survey. Men have smaller networks than women and tend to rely almost exclusively on their spouses. Both men and women prefer to provide more support than they receive; men tend to provide support to their spouse while women are more likely support friends and children. The only significant gender difference on measures of quality of support is men's report of greater marital satisfaction. For both sexes the quality of support has a greater influence on well-being than the quantity of support, but the quality and quantity of support have a greater effect on the well-being of women than men. [7.3, 7.5]

<458> Antonucci, T. C., & Akiyama, H. (1987). Social networks in adult life and a preliminary examination of the convoy model. *Journal of Gerontology, 42,* 519-527.

Investigates the social support networks for a national sample 718 older adults age 50-95, and examines the convoy of family and friends who surround the individual and help negotiate life's challenges. The average size of a network is nearly 9 members. Size or types of support receive do not differ by age. Older adults report more women than men as network members, about 57 percent women and 43 percent men. These findings indicate an active exchange of support among elderly adults, the presence of a convoy, and no gender differences in network size with aging. [7.5]

<459> Bosse, R., Aldwin, C. M., Levenson, M. R., Spiro, A. 3rd, & Mroczek, D. K. (1993). Change in social support after retirement: Longitudinal findings from the Normative Aging Study. *Journals of Gerontology: Psychological Sciences, 48,* P210-P217.

Studies the change in social support received after retirement among 1,311 men over a 3-year period. Although long-term retirees report the least amount of social support and continuing full-time workers the most, change in workforce status produced no apparent effect on quantity of support. Further, the quality of the support received shows no retirement effects. Findings affirm the distinction between retirement as a transition and retirement as a state. [7.5, 10.2]

<460> Bosse, R., Aldwin, C. M., Levenson, M. R., Workman-Daniels, K., & Ekerdt, D. J. (1990). Differences in social support among retirees and workers: Findings from the Normative Aging Study. *Psychology and Aging, 5,* 41-47.

Estimates the importance of coworkers as a sources of support in a sample of 1,513 older men. Half (56%) are working. Slightly fewer retirees than workers report coworker friends; long-term retirees report even fewer coworker friends. The greatest difference between retirees and workers is in type of support. Retirees almost never talked to former coworkers about problems they were having with retirement, finances, and marriage. Retirees' support gap is replaced by family and friends. Results support the notion of social support convoys, wherein coworkers constitute a component of the worker's convoy but decrease in importance as confidants retire. [7.5, 10.2]

<461> Bulcroft, K. A., Kielkopf, M. R., & Tripp, K. (1991). Elderly wards and their legal guardians: Analysis of county probate records in Ohio and Washington. *The Gerontologist, 31,* 156-164.

Evidence signals an increase in the use of legal guardianship in surrogate decision making for the elderly. Examines the profiles of older wards and their guardians, as well as the adjudication process experienced by older persons placed in legal guardianship. Finds more men than women are appointed guardians, contrary to the pattern where women are often designated as caregivers or case managers of older relatives. Contends that current statutes of guardianship may not be workable nor be fair to elders. Standardized and reliable assessments of competency are lacking, a family member's petition for guardianship is seldom challenged, and the primary goal of most guardianship cases is to preserve the estate. [7.5, 9.1, 9.2, 12.1]

<462> Chappell, N. L. (1991). In-group differences among elders living with friends and family other than spouses. *Journal of Aging Studies, 5,* 61-76.

Examines the characteristics of 431 elders who live with friends and family other than spouses. Finds support for a concept "independent elders"--those who live in their own household with either sisters or friends. Men are more likely to live with friends and women with siblings, and these "independent elders" are advantaged in terms of their socioeconomic status and/or health. Another group of "dependent elders" live within a married child's household, are disadvantaged in terms of both economics and health, and received considerable assistance from their married child. A third group consists of "traditional family relationships." Findings demonstrate the heterogeneity of consequences for those living with someone other than a spouse. [7.5, 11.2]

<463> Chappell, N. L. (1989). Health and helping among the elderly: Gender differences. *Journal of Aging and Health, 1,* 102-110.

Compares the helping networks of men and women in four different illness situations. Among 743 Canadians age 60 and older, networks vary depending on illness situation. Men more likely receive assistance from spouses and less likely from others. These gender patterns are evident only for less serious illness conditions. In the face of more serious health threats or functional limitations, gender differentials in spousal assistance disappear. These findings suggest that differential societal expectations for men and women dissipate in demanding health situations. [2.1, 7.5]

<464> Chatters, L. M., Taylor, R. J., & Jackson, J. S. (1986). Aged blacks' choices for an informal helper network. *Journal of Gerontology, 41,* 94-100.

Describes the relationships of sociodemographic, health, and family factors to choice of nine categories of helpers: spouse, son, daughter, father, mother, brother, sister, friend, and neighbor. Finds from logistic regression analysis that marital status is influential for the selection of sister, friend, and neighbor. Presence of children decreases the likelihood that siblings and friends are chosen. Family closeness facilitates the selection of siblings but inhibits the choice of friends. [7.5]

<465> Connidis, I. A., & Davis, L. (1992). Confidants and companions: Choices in later life. *Journals of Gerontology: Social Sciences, 47,* S115-S122.

Compares the correlates of a confidant or a companion being a spouse, child, sibling, other relative, or friend in a sample of 400 Canadians age 65 and older. Men and women are more similar than different as measured by the probability of their considering who is a confidant or companion. Men do report a smaller propensity to list children as companions and friends as confidants. There is evidence of substitution among the previously married and childless, with widowers substituting the loss of a spouse with children and friends for confiding, and children, friends, and other relatives for companionship. Geographical proximity is important for children's companionship and to confiding in siblings. Results correspond with studies using similar methods in Australia and the United States. [7.5]

<466> Depner, C. E., & Ingersoll-Dayton, B. (1988). Supportive relationships in later life. *Psychology and Aging, 3,* 348-357.

Examines four dimensions of the social support convoy of older adults: existence versus functioning of relationships, kinds of relationships (i.e., those with children, siblings, and friends), types of social support (i.e., emotional support, respect, and health support), and receipt versus provision of support. Using a national survey of 718 adults (age 50 and older), finds older people received less emotional and health support in the absence of sibling relationships. Otherwise, the effects of aging have more to do with what the older person contributes to the convoy than with what he or she receives. Men are less likely to include friends in their social support convoys, therefore women have better social support resources than men and receive more support from friends and children. No age and gender interaction is present, thus women's social support advantage does not counterbalance the effects of aging on the convoy. [7.5]

<467> Dorfman, L. T., & Mertens, C. E. (1990). Kinship relations in retired rural men and women. *Family Relations, 39,* 166-173.

Theorizes that retirement is a family experience as much as an individual one, and investigates the quantity and quality of intergenerational and sibling relationships for retired rural men (N = 252) and women (N = 199). The elders seem to be well integrated into kinship networks, although men are less involved in kinkeeping. Men receive less aid than females, as evidenced by proximity, frequency of contact, receipt of aid, and quality of relations (defined as affectional closeness and value consensus) with siblings and children. Overall satisfaction with family life is high for both men and women. [7.5, 8.1, 8.2, 10.2]

<468> Dwyer, J. W., Henretta, J. C., Coward, R. T., & Barton, A. J. (1992). Changes in the helping behaviors of adult children as caregivers. *Research on Aging, 14,* 351-375.

Reviews the prominent role of adult children in the care of older parents, particularly when the elder does not have a spouse, then describes changes in the caregiving responsibilities of the adult children over time. Data are from the 1982-1984 National Long-Term Care Survey. Adult children are 1.82 times more likely to have begun to provide ADL assistance when the elder was their mother than their father. [7.5, 9.2]

<469> Eggbeen, D. J. (1992). Family structure and intergenerational exchanges. *Research on Aging, 14,* 427-447.

Details the differentials in patterns of exchange of aid and assistance between elder parents and their non-coresidential children. Data are from the National Survey of Families and Households, and the overall levels of giving-receiving support between elder parents and adult children are not especially high. Older men receive markedly less money, assistance, and advice than women; they give less advice and childcare; they give more assistance and money. Divorced men are found to be significantly less likely than divorced women to give care or assistance to their children. [7.5, 10.1, 11.2]

<470> Felton, B. J., & Berry, C.A. (1992). Do the sources of the urban elderly's social support determine its psychological consequences? *Psychology & Aging, 7,* 89-97.

Studies the psychological effects of receiving different kinds of social support according to who provides it for 82 older adults. Hypothesizes the link between "social provisions" and emotional well-being vary when kin versus nonkin provide the support. Finds most social provisions are valuable regardless of their source. Reassurance of worth is distinctly more beneficial when provided by nonkin, and instrumental assistance is more strongly related to well-being when provided by kin. The social network structure shows that having duplicate providers for a given social provision is uniquely important in offsetting negative affect. [7.5]

<471> Ferraro, K. F., & Barresi, C, M. (1982). Impact of widowhood on the social relations of older persons. *Research on Aging, 4,* 227-247.

Examines longitudinally the impact of widowhood on elders' social relations. Data are from the National Survey of the Low-Income Aged and Disabled on 4,373 older marrieds and widowed. Widowhood did not immediately alter the older individual's quantity of interaction with family, friends, or neighbors. There is considerable familial continuity in the frequency of interaction for several years after the experience of widowhood for both men and women, and after 4 years decreases in family interaction are noticeable as interaction with neighbors increased. Widowers are not more socially isolated than widows. [7.1, 7.5]

<472> Ferraro, K. F., Mutran, E., & Barresi, C. M. (1984). Widowhood, health, and friendship support in later life. *Journal of Health and Social Behavior, 25,* 246-259.

Examines the effects of widowhood on the health and friendship support of older men and women. Data are from the 1973-1974 Survey of the Low-Income Aged and Disabled. Recently widowed elders evaluate their health more negatively than elders widowed for longer periods of time. Analysis of changes in friendship support show those widowed 1-4 years are more likely to increase their involvement in friendship. A multi-group analysis of married and widowed is also presented to examine if the causal processes affecting health and friendship support differ. Finds married and widowed older men are more likely to have friendship support than women, and being black is associated with more friendship support but poorer perceived health. [2.4, 7.5]

<473> Field, D., Winkler, M., Falk, R. F., & Leino, E. V. (1993). The influence of health on family contacts and family feelings in advanced old age: A longitudinal study. *Journals of Gerontology: Psychological Sciences, 48,* P18-P28.

Reports on a longitudinal analysis of the influences of health, age, gender, and socioeconomic status on family contacts and family feelings among 62 people age 74-

93. Primarily finds the stability of family contacts and feelings over the 14 year period, and as one moves through late life. Men express more satisfaction and involvement with families than women. Socioeconomic status declines in importance with advanced age. Working-class participants are initially more family focused, but with advanced age this class difference disappears for frequency of family contact, less so for feelings of satisfaction with families. Health increases in importance as a predictor. But rather than elders in poorer health, elders in greater health have greater family contact and feelings of closeness. It seems that in with advanced age, reciprocity between elders in good health is more central than socioeconomic status or gender. [2.1, 7.5, 8.2]

<474> Field, D., & Minkler, M. (1988). Continuity and change in social support between young-old and old-old or very-old age. *Journals of Gerontology: Psychological Sciences, 43*, P100-P106.

Longitudinally examines continuity and change in social support in a sample of 74 old-old (74 to 84) or very-old (85 and over) members of the Berkeley Older Generation Study. Considerable continuity in extent of contact is found for the group as a whole, particularly with respect to family relationships. In beyond-family contacts, declines are observed for men but not women, and for the very-old but not the old-old. Important changes are observed in involvement or subjective level of commitment: Satisfaction with children increased, while involvement beyond the family declined. [7.5]

<475> Johnson, C. L. (1983). Dyadic family relations and social support. *The Gerontologist, 23*, 377-383.

Presents findings from a study of the family support of 167 post-hospitalized elderly persons, examining how support varies by the relationship of the primary caregiver -- spouse, offspring, or another relative. The most comprehensive and unstressful support is provided by a spouse. In an analysis of the marital dyad, gender differences are apparent. Married female patients with husbands as caregivers have more frequent contact with children and other relatives, husband caregivers seek more help from formal caregivers, and husbands experience less strain, probably because secondary caregivers are present. Concludes that men prefer shared caregiving. [7.5, 8.4, 9.1]

<476> Keith, P. M. (1989). *The unmarried in later life*. New York: Praeger.

Examines being old and unmarried in the United States. Compares men and women who are single, formerly married or never married, and examines how differences in marital status affect older men's health and limitations, postponement of health care, finances, adaptations to retirement and loss of work, social participation and use of time. [7.5]

<477> Kendig, H. L., Coles, R., Pittelkow, Y., & Wilson, S. (1988). Confidants and family structure in old age. *Journals of Gerontology: Social Sciences, 43*, S31-S40.

Confiding has a major influence on well-being in old age, but little is known about the availability and selection of confidants. Using a survey of the social networks of 1,050 adults age 60 and older, this research explores the influence of age, gender, and family structure on choice of confidants. Except for the oldest age group, husbands are more likely than wives to confide in their spouse. Men and women report having an equal number of confidants, except in the oldest group where men have fewer. Findings support the premise that men are more dependent on intimacy within marriage than are women. [7.3, 7.5]

<478> Krause, N. (1991). **Stress and isolation from close ties in later life.** *Journals of Gerontology: Social Sciences, 46,* S183-S194.

Prior investigations of life stress and social support among older adults suggest that elders frequently cope with difficult times by turning to significant others. Evaluates an alternative view which suggests that particular stresses (financial strain, fear of crime) promote greater isolation. Data from 1,017 elders show that elders with chronic strain experience greater distrust, and distrust in turn leads to greater isolation from network members. The older men report less chronic strain from finances or fear of crime, but greater distrust of others and isolation from intimate ties than women. [2.3, 7.1, 7.5]

<479> Lee, G. R., Dwyer, J. W., & Coward, R. T. (1993). **Gender differences in parent care: Demographic factors and same-gender preferences.** *Journals of Gerontology: Social Sciences, 48,* S9-S16.

Tests the hypothesis that, when aging parents are assisted in the tasks of daily living by their adult children, the gender of the child providing the care depends in part on the gender of the parent receiving care. Data are on the 4,371 infirm elders from the National Long-Term Care Survey. Adult children are more likely to provide care for a parent of the same gender, and infirmed elders are more likely to receive care from a child of the same gender. Because the minority of elderly parents receiving care are fathers, this tendency toward gender consistency in caregiving partially accounts for the absence of sons in parent care. [7.5, 8.2, 9.1]

<480> Lund, D. A., Caserta, M. S., Van Pelt, J., & Gass, K. A. (1990). **Stability of social support after later-life spousal bereavement.** *Death Studies, 14,* 53-73.

Investigates the degree of stability in the structural and qualitative aspects of the social support networks of 108 bereaved spouses between ages 50 and 89. The primary network for bereaved men and women include 8-9 people, yet men have fewer contacts with members than women, and the number of contacts decreases over the first two years of bereavement. The size of men's secondary network, although initially small, increases significantly over time, to a point where it exceeds women's. Among the men age 75 and older, the networks are as gender homogeneous as women's. [7.5]

<481> Markides, K. S., Boldt, J. S., & Ray, L. A. (1986). **Sources of helping and intergenerational solidarity: A three-generation study of Mexican Americans.** *Journal of Gerontology, 41,* 506-511.

Studies the degree of intergenerational solidarity and sources of help and advice in a three-generation sample of Mexican Americans. Elderly Mexican Americans are involved in strong helping networks with their children, who rely on the elders. Finds older men are relied on for home repairs and upkeep, and older women are depended on for health matters. Seeking advice and help regarding finances and personal problems is not done across sex--adult sons consult elder fathers. All-female dyads have greater intergenerational solidarity than all male and cross-sex dyads, and there appears to be minimum intergenerational helping between grandparents and grandchildren. [7.5, 8.2]

<482> Miller, B., & McFall, S. (1991). Stability and change in the informal task support network of frail older persons. *The Gerontologist, 31*, 735-745.

Recognizes the importance of the stability of the informal care network to elder and community well-being. Investigates what predicts stability in composition, size, and intensity of help within frail elders' support networks. Data are from the 1982 and 1984 National Long-Term Care Surveys (N = 940 and 644) and reveal elders receive help from more than one helper. Those who are married, male, white and more educated have fewer helpers, however networks consisting only of a spouse or adult child provide more assistance proportionate to their size than other networks. There is relative stability in the composition and size of support networks. Changes in network size and intensity of help occur in response to changes in health and functional status of the frail older person, particularly for black Americans. Blacks larger networks may reflect the social convoy model of providing support. [7.5, 9.1]

<483> Miller, B., McFall, S., & Cambell, R. T. (1994). Changes in sources of community long-term care among African American and white frail older persons. *Journals of Gerontology: Social Sciences, 49*, S14-S24.

Examines longitudinally race differences among older persons' changes in sources of long-term care. Using data from the 1982-84 National Long-Term Care Survey, in the 2-year period whites are less likely to be deceased, less likely to rely solely on informal helpers, and more likely to be institutionalized. Findings also show that frail white men are about twice as likely to have acquired formal and informal help as the frail white women, and African American men are more, but not significantly more likely than African American women to have added informal and/or formal help. [7.5, 12.3]

<484> Pearlman, D. N., & Crown, W. H. (1992). Alternative sources of social support and their impacts on institutional risk. *The Gerontologist, 32*, 527-535.

Examines longitudinally the direct and buffering effects of different dimensions of social support on the risk of being institutionalized over a two-year period. Multivariate analyses indicate that specific aspects of social support, such as having a spouse or adult child caregiver, or having a longer (at least 3 years) caregiving relationship, buffer the stress of being dependent on others for care and the outcome of institutionalization. While no direct gender differences are noted, networks that include a paid provider (which are common among older husbands) modestly offset the impact of the frail elder's impairment on admission to a nursing home. [7.5, 11.2]

<485> Perry, C. M., & Johnson, C. L. (1994). **Families and support networks among African American oldest-old.** *International Journal of Aging and Human Development, 38,* 41-50.

Determines the social networks available to the oldest-old. The sample consists of 122 (26 men and 96 women) community-dwelling African Americans age 85 and older who are administered the same interview protocol as the 150 whites in the San Francisco 85+ Study. Marital status and living arrangements show men are more often married (38 percent versus 8 percent of women) and not living alone (65 percent versus 33 percent). Only a minority of the men and women receive instrumental help from a child on a regular basis, and even fewer receive such assistance from relatives. Results suggests that unmarried and childless men may be at risk for social isolation and a compromised quality of life. These findings support the view that oldest-old blacks are a heterogeneous group whose family structure mirrors that of younger-old groups. [7.5]

<486> Rubinstein, R. L. (1987). **Never married elderly as a social type: Re-evaluating some images.** *The Gerontologist, 27,* 108-113.

Stereotypes about the never married elderly are assessed from two studies. In one, 47 older men living alone (11 never married) are interviewed; in the other, the well-being and social ties and relations of 34 never married men in a larger study of community-resident elderly are examined. The studies reveal that never married men live in varied social and coresidential circumstances, and that many have social networks containing members who are subjectively close. Loneliness is a problem for some, but not all, of the respondents. It is concluded that not all the never married elderly fulfill the characteristics of a single "social type." [2.1, 7.5]

<487> Silverstein, M., & Waite, L. J. (1993). **Are blacks more likely than whites to receive and provide social support in middle and old age? Yes, no, and maybe so.** *Journals of Gerontology: Social Sciences, 48,* S212-S222.

Investigates differences in the social support exchanges of white and black men and women from mid-life to old age using data from the 1987-88 National Survey of Families and Households. Black men are less likely than white men to provide and receive instrumental support, and no more or less likely to provide emotional support. Black-white differences in three comparisons are generally consistent over the age range among men, providing little evidence of a contextual effect of age. Older white men provide no more or less emotional support but receive less than older black men. Older men tend to provide as much instrumental assistance as emotional (but as gender socialization would predict, somewhat less than older women provide). [7.5]

<488> Spitze, G., & Logan, J. R. (1989). **Gender differences in family support: Is there a payoff?** *The Gerontologist, 29,* 108-113.

Studies of parent-child contact and assistance concentrate on gender differences in the children's generation, not between parents. Data from a national sample of adults over age 65 reveals that, men are more likely to be living with a spouse. Overall, men live further from children and have marginally less contact, receive fewer telephone calls, but no less mail than women. Men who live alone receive slightly fewer visits and assistance. Men's receipt of less informal assistance is explained by lessor need levels.

These findings provide little to no evidence that men's prior lack of kinkeeping yields less contact in old age. [7.5, 9.1, 11.2]

<489> Stoller, E. P., Forster, L. E., & Duniho, T. S. (1992). Systems of parent care within sibling networks. *Research on Aging, 14*, 28-49.

Examines what factors explain the participation of adult children, what factors influence the selection of the primary helper, and what factors explain the selection of a son as primary helper. From a sample of 753 elders age 65 and over from upstate New York, finds the presence of a proximate child is the only significant predictor of the adult child being included in the parent's helping network and named primary helper. The availability of a proximate son increases his likelihood of being named the primary helper, especially when there are few proximate daughters. Widowed fathers show no preference, and fathers who are no longer married are more likely to name siblings and friends as helpers. [7.5, 8.2, 9.1]

<490> Taylor, R. J. (1985). The extended family as a source of support to elderly blacks. *The Gerontologist, 25*, 488-495.

Examines the influence of family and demographic factors on the frequency of support received from family members among a sample of 581 blacks age 55 and older. Finds men receive family support much less than women, and these findings parallel prior investigations of white elders. The consistency of the gender difference suggest that men do less kin-keeping and are less affiliated and connected to their families, perhaps regardless of age in the life-span. [7.5, 9.1]

<491> Taylor, R. J., & Chatters, L. M. (1986). Patterns of informal support to elderly black adults: Family, friends, and church members. *Social Work, 31*, 432-438.

Data are from the National Survey of Black Americans, and are used to describe the sources of support for the 581 elderly blacks age 55 or older. The extent and types of family, friends, and non-kin (e.g., church) support perceived to be available are profiled. Eight of ten elders report they receive support from a best or close friend and from church members, and half receive support from family members. Families provide more material support and friends more companionship. [7.5]

<492> Taylor, R. J., & Chatters, L. M. (1986). Church-based informal support among elderly blacks. *The Gerontologist, 26*, 637-642.

Analyzes data from the National Survey of Black Americans to examine the receipt of church-based support. Both frequency and amount of support are predicted by frequency of church attendance. Socioemotional support during illness is the most prevalent form of reported aid. [2.3, 7.5]

<493> Taylor, R. J., & Chatters, L. M. (1991). Extended family networks of older black adults. *Journals of Gerontology: Social Sciences, 46*, S210-S217.

Three characteristics of familial networks--residential proximity, family affection, and family contact--among elder black Americans are described. The proximity of an adult child and of relatives facilitates emotional and social integration of elders in family networks. Greater interaction and stronger emotional bonds are noted for older blacks and their extended families. No age differences in levels of contact and emotional closeness are observed. [7.5]

<494> Van Tilburg, T. (1992). Support networks before and after retirement. *Journal of Social and Personal Relationships, 9,* **433-445.**

Examines alterations in the support networks of 50 men (age 55-65) before and after retirement. The men are interviewed just before retirement and again one year later. Changes occur in the form of their networks: Although the size remains stable, the composition of the network changes dramatically. Many relationships, especially those with colleagues, are terminated. The functions of the networks undergo changes such that more support is given and the reciprocity of the networks decreases. However, reciprocity is a factor in the continuation of relationships. Reciprocal relationships have a greater chance of continuation, and "overbenefiting" relationships are more often terminated than are "underbenefiting" relationships. [7.5]

<495> Whitbeck, L., Hoyt, D. R., & Huck, S. M. (1994). Early family relationships, intergenerational solidarity, and support provided to parents by their adult children. *Journals of Gerontology: Social Sciences, 49,* **S85-S94.**

Investigates the effects of early family experiences on the quality of the adult child-parent relationship, and on the extent of instrumental and emotional support provided elderly parents by their children. Based on adult children's reports regarding 1,135 aging parents, the propensity to offer aging fathers and mothers instrumental and emotional support is indirectly affected by the influence of the early parent-child relationship. Fathers' early rejection (i.e., fault-finding, blame) negatively affects children's filial concern and is associated with a strained contemporary relationship. Both of these are directly related to less support. [7.5, 8.2]

<496> Wilcox, V. L., Kasl, S. V., & Berkman, L. F. (1994). Social support and physical disability in older people after hospitalization: A prospective study. *Health Psychology, 13,* **170-179.**

Examines prospectively the effects of social support on recovery from physical disability among 84 hip fracture, 79 stroke, and 106 myocardial infarction elders identified at hospitalization. Illness precipitates changes in both the qualitative and quantitative aspects of social support, mobilizing support for some individuals and leaving others with no one. The number of emotional support providers and the adequacy of task support are higher after hospitalization, yet the adequacy of emotion support is poorer and the percentage of people reporting "no one to count on" increases. Believing that one can handle the emotional demands of illness without assistance predicts better functional outcomes than needing and receiving emotional support. [7.5]

8

Family Relations

— ◆ —

SIBLINGS

<497> Cicirelli, V. G. (1977). Relationships of siblings to the elderly person's feelings and concerns. *Journal of Gerontology, 32,* 317-322.

A projective instrument reveals the feelings and concerns of elderly persons in relation to the number and sex of their siblings. Partial correlations, with effects of age, education, and occupation removed, are computed separately for each sex. The number and proportion of female siblings are found to have a greater influence than male siblings. For men, sister siblings are more emotionally supportive. [7.5, 8.1]

<498> Connidis, I. A. (1989). Siblings as friends in later life. *American Behavioral Scientist, 33,* 81-93.

Examines the role of siblings as friends in elders' lives. Affirms several assumptions in the literature about siblings, and fails to substantiate others. The most obvious contradiction is the lack of association between gender and siblings being close friends or mutual confidants. Brothers or brother-sister dyads are no less close than sisters. Siblings who are unmarried are inclined to seek out closeness (confiding, geographic proximity) more than married siblings. [8.1]

<499> Connidis, I. A. (1994). Sibling support in older age. *Journal of Gerontology: Social Sciences, 49,* S309-S317.

Only a minority of the 528 men and women age 55 and over in the sample receive any of the instrumental forms of help from a sibling (i.e., help when ill, financial assistance, other instrumental help). At most, one-quarter received such help. The gender characteristics of the relationship between siblings indicate that men with a sister are least likely to receive support when ill, followed by men with a brother, and then women with a brother. Men with a sibling of either gender are less likely to report receipt of help when sick. For both men and women, there is a greater likelihood of aid from a sibling of the same sex. Nonetheless, people feel their siblings are available, and siblings are an important perceived "insurance policy" in later life. [7.5, 8.1, 9.2]

<500> Gold, D. T. (1989). Generational solidarity: Conceptual antecedents and consequences. *American Behavioral Scientist, 33,* 19-32.

Examines in a two-year longitudinal study sibling relationships across the life course for 54 men and women age 67-89. Eight constructs describe sibling relationships: closeness, envy, resentment, instrumental support, emotional support, psychological involvement, acceptance/approval, and contact. Two dimensions remain unchanged over time -- closeness and contact. Despite not feeling closer or having any more contact, siblings report thinking about their brothers and sisters more frequently and experiencing deeper feelings of acceptance and approval. Men have less contact and closeness and fewer support exchanges, and they have greater feelings of resentment and lower levels of acceptance (approval) with their brothers. Late-life sibling relationships are not uniformly static or dynamic, the majority are positively oriented in quality and meaning, and are built more on shared history or "generational solidarity." [8.1]

<501> Gold, D. T. (1989). Sibling relationships in old age: A typology. *International Journal of Aging and Human Development, 28,* 37-51.

Recognizes that sibling interaction in old age has received limited attention. Examines the ways in which different kinds of relationships between siblings in old age meet or ignore the social and psychological needs of the older people. The typology identifies five types of sibling relationships (intimate, congenial, loyal, apathetic, hostile) from data collected in interviews with 30 men and 30 women age 65 and older. Each type reflects a discrete pattern of instrumental and emotional support, contact, closeness, envy, resentment, approval, and involvement with the sibling. Gender of the respondent does not influence the kinds of relationship that exists. But, dyads involving a sister are distributed more heavily in the intimate and congenial types than are brother-brother dyads. Sibling interaction seems based on gender composition of the dyad rather than the gender of the respondent. When the dyad involves a sister, there is greater psychological involvement and attachment. [8.1]

<502> Gold, D. T. (1990). Late-life sibling relationships: Does race affect typological distribution? *The Gerontologist, 30,* 741-748.

Studies the effects of race on characteristics of late-life sibling relations. Race does have an effect on sibling dyads, and the distribution of black sibling pairs is skewed toward the positive categories -- intimate, congenial, and loyal. White dyads cover the spectrum and some are apathetic or hostile. Older black brothers and sisters report more positive attitudes toward their siblings and show greater interest in providing support. Using log linear models, only those dyadic gender combinations that include men (i.e., male-male and male-female dyads) significantly differ by race. [8.1]

<503> Gold, D. T., Woodbury, M. A., & George, L. K. (1990). Relationship classification using grade of membership analysis: A typology of sibling relationships in later life. *Journals of Gerontology: Social Sciences, 45,* S43-S51.

Compares two typologies of sibling relationships in later life, one based on constant comparative analysis, a qualitative technique, and the other based on the grade of membership procedure which combines qualitative and quantitative analyses. Data are the key words, phrases, and metaphorical language of 30 older men and 30 older women. Four pure types of relationships involving five behavioral and emotional dimensions are identified, but two dimensions (apathy and hostility) may not be meaningfully different. Moderate closeness, psychological involvement, and support, without feelings of envy or resentment, characterize cross-sex siblings. Older men's relationships with sisters and, particularly, with brothers are just as likely to be characterized by low closeness and involvement, with modest envy and instrumental support, or by no psychological involvement, support, but feelings of rejection. [1.3, 8.1]

<504> Matthews, S. H., Delaney, P. J., & Adamek, M. E. (1989). Male kinship ties: Bonds between adult brothers. *American Behavioral Scientist, 33,* 58-69.

Bonds between brothers virtually have been ignored. The authors examine 49 sibling relationships involving brothers who have no sisters and whose parents are in the empty nest or widowhood stage of the life cycle. Without the influence of a sister, who might act as a kinkeeper of the sibling group, the question is in what ways are older brothers involved in one another's lives. Four levels of affiliation are identified--closely affiliated, lukewarm, disaffiliated, or disparate. Geographic proximity is not related to level of affiliation in a straightforward way, but brothers closer in age and continuously married are more closely affiliated. Findings affirm the possibility that brothers use different vocabularies to talk about feelings for one another. [1.1, 8.1]

<505> Matthews, S. H. (1994). Men's ties to siblings in old age: Contributing factors to availability and quality. In E. Thompson (Ed.), *Older men's lives* (pp. 178-196). Thousand Oaks, CA: Sage Publications.

Begins asking not whether there is variation, but what is the best way to describe it in sibling relationships. Uses qualitative data from the Older Families Study and gender as a theoretically central construct to examine the how men's and women's lives influence siblings bonds in later life. Recognizes the disadvantage men face with researchers' expectations that older men care less about relationships than women and are not able to talk about them. Although men's descriptions of sibling relations might seem less "rich," their lives are more embedded in marriages and families of procreation, thus perhaps their sibling relations are more constricted. Concludes urging researchers to appreciate how gender and other variables outside individuals pattern sibling ties of older men. [8.1]

<506> Spitze, G., & Logan, J. R. (1991). Sibling structure and intergenerational relations. *Journal of Marriage and the Family, 53,* 871-884.

Examines effects of adults siblings' number, gender, and birth order on their relationships with parents. Sibling structure does not affect children's closeness to parents or attitudes about filial responsibilities, however the number of siblings does reduce contact and helping. The results from the two data sources--the adult child's perspective and then the parent's perspective--on visiting, telephone contacts, and helping are not fully consistent. Concludes that when older parents are interviewed, they report relations with children as being more similar, in closeness and in frequency, than they actually are. [8.1, 8.2]

FATHERHOOD AND FAMILY TIES

<507> Bulcroft, K. A., & Bulcroft, R. A. (1991). The timing of divorce: Effects on parent-child relationships in later life. *Research on Aging, 13*, 226-243.

Assesses the effects of marital status on contact with adult children. Data are from the National Survey of Families and Households. Finds, as hypothesized, divorce has a negative effect on interaction with adult children, and this effect is much greater for men than for women. Men who divorced when their children were young have the lowest rates of interaction, suggesting the long-term consequences of divorce for men are particularly deleterious for interaction with their children. Although inconclusive, filial responsibility norms seem to vary by family type and may be quite low for children of noncustodial fathers. [8.2]

<508> Burton, L. M., & Dilworth-Anderson, P. (1991). The intergenerational family roles of aged Black Americans. *Marriage and Family Review, 16*, 311-330.

Examines the literature on the intergenerational family roles of elderly black men and women. This discussion addresses roles created by vertical ties in families--between aged parents and adult children, grandparents and grandchildren, and older family members and extended kin. Available research on the black elderly as aged parents, grandparents, and kin-keepers in extended kin networks is spare. [1.4, 8.2, 8.3]

<509> Greenberg, J. S., & Becker, M. (1988). Aging parents as family resources. *The Gerontologist, 28*, 786-791.

Contends that researchers have all but ignored the role of aging parents as family resources. Examines the extent to which aging parents experience stress when problems arise in the lives of their adult children, and the ways in which they serve as resources to their children in need. For older couples, fathers and mothers experience high levels of stress as a result of their adult children's problems. For fathers, distress is not directly correlated with the stress experienced by the adult children, rather it appears affected by their wives' distress with the children's problems. Son's dependence is particularly stressful for fathers. All elder parents are actively helping their children cope. [8.2]

<510> Hernandez, G. G. (1992). The family and its aged members: The Cuban experience. *Clinical Gerontologist, 11* (3/4), 45-57.

Discusses the role of gender and family ties to Cubans' experience of aging. Calls attention to their cultural and historical experiences, and identified as pivotal their African heritage, hierarchical structure of the family, and religion. Specific recommendations with regard to gender are provided to clinicians working with Cuban families with aged members, such as the need to not mix older men and women when creating support groups, because the group will become a social group with men controlling group activities and it will not produce therapeutic results. [7.5, 8.2]

<511> Kimmel, D. C. (1992). Families of older gay men and lesbians. *Generations, 17* (3), 37-38.

Describes different types of family relationships of older gay men (and lesbians). Many may be involved in a long-term relationship, which are more frequent than is commonly assumed. Older gays typically live within a self-created network of friends, significant others, and selected biological family members, and the network provides mutual support of various kinds, just as a family system might do. Some men have special roles in their family of origin that reflect their unique social position--they may be caretakers of aging relatives, "selected" for the job because of being unmarried or geographically mobile. Concludes by calling attention to the significance of group differences in aging. [1.1, 7.3, 8.2, 9.1]

<512> Lawton, L., Silverstein, M., & Bengtson, V. L. (1994). Affection, social contact, and geographic distance between adult children and their parents. *Journal of Marriage and the Family, 56,* 57-68.

Investigates whether greater affection between adult children and their patients leads to more social contact, whether frequent contact leads to greater affection, or whether each of these mutually influences the other. From a 1990 sample collected by the American Association of Retired Persons, reciprocal effects are not observed in the father-child relationship. Fondness for older fathers does not translate into greater familiarity. Motivations for contact with fathers are more instrumental and less personal affinity, and the decision to socialize tends not to be made by the father. Parental divorce markedly diminishes frequency of contact with the father, thus structural and personal features are fitting to understand parent-child relations in later life. [8.2]

<513> Peterson, C. C., & Peterson, J. L. (1988). Older men's and women's relationships with adult kin: How equitable are they? *International Journal of Aging and Human Development, 27,* 221-231.

Extends research on equity perceptions to 62 elderly men's and women's relationships with their spouses, adult children, and aged parents. A comparison group of 40 younger adults also rates the equity of their marriages and relationships with elder parents and grandparents. The majority of elderly men's and women's involvement with all categories of immediate adult kin are distinguished by strict global equity--or, a balanced set of gains and losses accruing from the interaction together. Comments how the equity finding is somewhat surprising, given a lifetime's experience in the equity equation. Most departures from strict equity involve feeling subjectively overbenefited rather than under-benefited. For example, young adults fell greater relative benefit from their fathers and mothers than older fathers and mothers subjectively gain from their adults sons and daughters. [8.2, 8.4]

<514> Pett, M. A., Lang, N., & Gander, A. (1992). Late-life divorce. *Journal of Family Issues, 13,* 526-552.

Examines the impact of late-life divorce on family rituals in interviews with 73 women and 42 men who are the children of 111 divorced older persons. As reported, older parents' divorce requires years of renegotiation and restructuring of tasks, composition, and boundaries. Some of the family rituals are maintained, and others are irrevocably changed with new rituals constructed from old ones. A strong association is found between perceived disruptiveness of the parental divorce and changes in family rituals, particularly at Thanksgiving and Christmas. [8.2, 8.4]

<515> Seccombe, K.   (1988).   Financial assistance from elderly retirement-age sons to their aging parents. *Research on Aging, 10,* 102-118.

Contributes to the understanding of intergenerational caregiving by exploring the exchange of financial aid between elderly sons and the oldest old. Using data from the Retirement History Longitudinal Survey, one out of every eight retirement-age sons reports providing financial aid to an aging parent. Among caregiving tasks, financial assistance is a rare event among elderly children. Frequency of interaction between generations is the strongest predictor of exchange of aid from son to parent. [8.2, 9.1]

<516> Silverstein, M., & Litwak, E.   (1993).   A task-specific typology of inter-generational family structure in later life. *The Gerontologist, 33,* 258-264.

Uses a model of intergenerational social support to analyze data from 910 dyads of older adults and their primary child helpers. The results argue against the unidimensionality of intergenerational social support. Social-emotional support is contingent on the quality of the dyadic relationship and personal affinity. This type of support is provided regardless of parents' physical functioning or presence of a spouse. It is more a "normal" aspect of family functioning. However, task support is contingent on elder health and structural conditions--the gender of parent, adult child's unmarried status, and geographic distance between the generations. Older fathers are more likely in a modified-extended support relationship than a traditional one, reflecting how fathers are less often the primary exchange parent with adult children. [7.5, 8.2, 8.4]

<517> Speare, A., & Avery, R.   (1993).   Who helps whom in older parent-child families. *Journals of Gerontology: Social Sciences, 48,* S64-S73.

Previous research assumes that older persons who live with adult children do so because of the poverty or disability, but recent evidence suggests that many of these extended households primarily benefit the child. Data from the Survey of Income and Program Participation reveal that coresidence becomes less likely with parent age. Older fathers are less likely to be living with children when age and other factors are controlled. When children live with parents under age 75, they are likely to be the primary beneficiaries of the relationship. [8.2]

<518> Spitze, G., & Miner, S.   (1992).   Gender differences in adult child contact among black elderly parents. *The Gerontologist, 32,* 213-218.

Examines gender differences in levels of contact with children and the determinants of that contract. Data are on 575 black middle-aged and elderly parents from a national probability sample. Men, especially those who live alone, experience substantially less child contact--fewer visits and phone calls per year--than do women. This pattern is not explained by fathers' needs, resources, or child availability. Black fathers' potential isolation, at least from children, may be partly choice. [8.2]

<519> Spitze, G., & Logan, J. R. (1992). **Helping as a component of parent-adult child relations.** *Research on Aging, 14,* 291-312.

Examines the patterns of helping between parents and their adult children. Focuses on the frequency of several types of help provided in both directions between parents and adult children over the life course. Finds parental help to children is the norm, rather than the reverse, until parents reach age 75. Gendered patterns of helping are evident, but in contrast to expectations, there is no consistent pattern of helping among gender-pairs. One-third of the fathers regularly help sons, but more fathers help daughters for slightly fewer hours per week. Effects of gender do not disappear when other factors are controlled. Both daughter-father and son-father pairs involve significantly less help to the parent than for mother pairs. [8.2]

<520> Thomas, J. L. (1994). **Older men as fathers and grandfathers.** In E. Thompson (Ed.), *Older men's lives* (pp. 197-217). Thousand Oaks, CA: Sage Publications.

Using a contextual approach where individual relationships are nodes in an elaborate family network and reflections of the cultural setting, this chapter systematically reviews the available research on older men as fathers in the launching stage and the reorganization which follows in types and frequency of contact with adult children, feelings of affection, and support exchanges. Defines as long overdue research which explicitly considers fatherhood in late adulthood. Concludes with a discussion of the future directions for research, including meta-analytic studies of family roles for older men's well-being. Emphasizes need to move beyond descriptive work to thoroughly examine older men's experiences as fathers and grandfathers. [8.2, 8.3]

<521> Troll, L. E. (1987). **Gender differences in cross-generation networks.** *Sex Roles, 17,* 751-766.

Reviews the literature on gender differences in parent-child relationships in later life, and argues that kin networks tend to have an integrity of their own. Help from one generation to another is reciprocal over life, shifting from the younger generation to the older generation as circumstances change. However, neither aid nor contact are pre-dictive of intimacy. The grandfather-son-grandson line appears to be almost as impor-tant as the grandmother-mother-granddaughter line, with male members of the line trying to influence each other over career and nonfamily matters, while female members providing advice on interpersonal and intrafamily matters. Men and women both tend to be less involved with older fathers than with older mothers or in-laws. Concludes that the literature contains problems of conceptualization and measurement, including ambiguous definitions of constructs such as closeness and affect. [8.2, 8.3]

GRANDFATHERHOOD

<522> Boxer, A. M., Cook, J. A., & Cohler, B. J. (1986). **Grandfathers, fathers, and sons: Intergenerational relations among men.** In K. A. Pillemer and R. S. Wolf (Eds.), *Elder abuse: Conflict in the family* (pp. 93-121). Dover, MA: Auburn House.

Prior research on men's intergenerational relations notes that men often have difficulty expressing feelings of closeness to other men. Studies conflict among three generations of men (young adults, middle-aged fathers, and grandfathers), finds the man's position in the generational hierarchy affects male-to-male ties. Grandfathers perceive the least conflict in relations with their sons and grandsons and use avoidance to deal with conflict. Men's family relationships are more diverse and less homogeneous than previously recognized, and they are influenced both by the vertical position in the family and the position in the life course. Use of a female model of family relations should be avoided in studying men's intergenerational ties. [8.2, 8.3]

<523> Forsyth, C. J., Roberts, S. B., & Robin, C. A. (1992). Variables influencing life satisfaction among grandparents. *International Journal of Sociology and the Family, 22*, 51-60.

Analyzes the sources of life satisfaction among 252 grandparents. Factors affecting life satisfaction are investigated regressing eleven predictors (e.g., sociodemographic, health, interaction with grandchildren). Gender has a significant effect on the level of life satisfaction experienced, with men reporting less life satisfaction. [2.3, 8.3]

<524> Johnson, C. L., & Barer, B. M. (1987). Marital instability and the changing kinship networks of grandparents. *The Gerontologist, 27*, 330-335.

Introduces how the incidence of divorce and remarriage has made marked changes on families and kinship reorganization. Examines how organizational changes in kinship change kinship networks of grandparents. Using a sample of white, middle-class families, three years after the divorces of children, half of the networks of the older generations expand. A common source of expansion is among paternal grandmothers who retain relationships with their former daughters-in-law and her relatives at the same time that they added new relatives with their sons' remarriages. [8.3]

<525> Hodgson, L. G. (1992). Adult grandchildren and their grandparents: The enduring bond. *International Journal of Aging & Human Development, 34*, 209-225.

Offers an understanding of the often unnoticed family role--the adult grandchild. From a national survey of 208 adult grandchildren, the strength of the bonds--the levels of contact and perceptions of closeness--between grandchildren and the "closest" grandparent are examined. For the two dimensions, the bonds in relationships are significant and meaningful. Levels of contact are generally high, and most grandchildren report that their relationships with grandparents are enduring. Related to the strength of the adult grandchild-grandparent bonds are matriarchal lineage, geographical proximity, and the earlier child/parent relationship. [8.3]

<526> Kennedy, G. E. (1990). College students' expectations of grandparent and grandchild role behaviors. *The Gerontologist, 30*, 43-48.

Examines the attitudes of 704 college students toward their grandparents and the grandparent role. Grandparent/grandchild constellations ranged from students with eight or more grandparents to those with no living grandparent. Students tend to feel less close to their father's parents than to their mother's and are closer to grandmothers than to grandfathers. [8.3]

<527> Kennedy, G. E. (1992). Quality of grandparent/grandchild relationships. *International Journal of Aging and Human Development, 35*, 83-98.

Prior work suggests elements of quality can be identified for the grandparent/grandchild relationship. Examines 391 young adults' perceptions of the quality of their relationships with their "most close" grandparent. Grandsons more than granddaughters identify grandfathers as their most-close grandparent, yet grandfathers are one-half as likely to be the most-close grandparent. Two-thirds of the most-close grandparents are grandmothers, which reflects longevity effects on opportunity, styles of relating to grandchildren, and frequency of one-on-one contact. [8.3]

<528> Kivett, V. R. (1985). Grandfathers and grandchildren: Patterns of association, helping, and psychological closeness. *Family Relations, 34*, 565-571.

Studies 99 grandfathers living in a rural transitional area. Compared with other late life roles, the grandfatherhood is of little relative importance to the older men. It is subordinate to other family roles. There is some evidence of a continuing level of contact between most older men and at least one grandchild, and proximity is the factor most consistently related to a relationship. The moderate to low levels of interaction between grandfathers and grandchildren and limited mutual assistance indicate interaction is most often restricted to ceremony and rituals. Yet, grandfathers perceive more closeness than others would find and expect assistance in the event of adversity. [7.5, 8.3]

<529> Kivett, V. (1991). The grandparent-grandchild connection. *Marriage and Family Review, 16* (3-4), 267-290.

Summarizes information on gender differences in the grandparent-grandchild connection. Patterns show the relative unimportance of men's roles in family life compared to those of women's -- grandchildren are more involved with maternal than paternal grandparents, and grandfathers provide more instrumental and less expressive relationships. Differences in grandparenting might be expected between current cohorts of middle aged and older adults given their family/work involvements and differences in gender ideologies. [8.3]

<530> Oyserman, D., Radin, N., & Benn, R. (1993). Dynamics in a three-generational family: Teens, grandparents, and babies. *Developmental Psychology, 29*, 564-572.

Tests the hypotheses that grandmothers have a direct influence on their teenage grandchild, and grandparents have an indirect effect on the teenager's young child through their influence on the teen's nurturance and her perceptions of family support. Data are from a sample of 64 working-class families with two-grandparents and a teen and her child. Major findings are that grandfathers had a direct effect on children and that grandmothers had neither direct nor indirect influence. These results are discussed in terms of the salience of nurturant grandfathers in these families and the unique role they may play in the family. [8.3]

<531> **Roberto, K. A., & Stroes, J.   (1992).   Grandchildren and grandparents: Roles, influences, and relationships.** *International Journal of Aging and Human Development, 34,* **227-239.**

Uses a sample of 142 college students to explore the significance of grandparents in the lives of young adult grandchildren. The grandchildren report that they participate in more activities with grandmothers than grandfathers--particularly brief visits for conversation or talking over things that are important. Grandfathers are, in turn, perceived as having less influence in the students' value development than grandmothers, and the strength of the grandfather/grandchild relationship is not as strong as the one between grandmother and grandchild. Discusses how conventional gender beliefs influence perception of grandparents, and grandfathers in particular, defining what constitutes appropriate domains of conversation and who to turn to when interpersonal issues are the concern. [8.3]

<532> **Russell, G.   (1986).   Grandfathers: Making up for lost opportunities. In R. A. Lewis and R. E. Salt (Eds.),** *Men in families* **(pp. 233-259). Beverly Hills, CA: Sage Publications.**

Explores the experience of grandfathering, as described by parents with young children and the maternal and paternal grandparents from the same family systems. The 32 grandfathers derive considerable satisfaction from grandparenting and rate it as a highly significant aspect of their lives. Most are highly active in when they saw their grandchildren. They tend to participate more in physical and outdoor activities than conventional play. Grandfathers give high priority to the pride and joy that accompanies grandparenting, and to being available to their adult children in times of social and financial need. Paternal grandfathers spend less time with their grandchildren than maternal grandfathers, and they are more traditional in their interactions, but they rate the quality of their relationships with their grandchildren just as highly as maternal grandfathers. Many grandfathers consider grandparenting as an opportunity to compensate for what they perceive as insufficient involvement with their own children. [8.3]

<533> **Strom, R., Collinsworth, P., Strom, S., & Griswold, D. (1992-93). Strengths and needs of black grandparents.** *International Journal of Aging and Human Development, 36,* **255-268.**

Examines ethnic differences in grandparent performance and effectiveness through the perceptions of 204 white and 204 black grandparents and 175 white and 295 black grandchildren. Black grandparents perceive themselves more favorably than did whites on all six subscales tapping grandparent strengths and needs. In multivariate analysis, gender never emerges to show a main or interactive effect. Rather, significant main effects are observed for ethnicity and age of grandparent, age of grandchild, time spent together, and geographical proximity. [8.3]

<534> **Thomas, J. L. (1986). Age and sex differences in perceptions of grandparenting.** *Journal of Gerontology, 41,* **417-423.**

Describes relationships between grandparents' age and sex and grandparenting satisfaction and perceive responsibilities. Data from 277 grandparents in three age groups
reveal that grandfathers in general and the younger grandparents express greater
responsibility for caretaking and offering childrearing advice, but less satisfaction with
grandparenting. When number of grandchildren and their ages are controlled, grandfathers express greater responsibility for offering childrearing advice and caretaking, but
report less satisfaction with grandparenting. [8.3]

<535> Thomas, J. L. (1986). **Gender differences in satisfaction with grandparent-
ing.** *Psychology and Aging, 1,* 215-219.

Although gender differences in family experiences are studied, grandmothers and
grandfathers are rarely compared. White grandfathers (N = 105) and grandmothers (N
= 177) provide information on their grandparenting satisfaction and perceived respon-
sibilities--disciplining, caretaking, helping, advising. Although the importance of gender
is small and not overwhelming, differences are noted. Grandfathers' satisfaction scores
are exceeded by those of grandmothers in three of five domains, however grandmothers' greater satisfaction scores seem to reflect continuity of earlier family experiences and grandmothers older age. [8.3]

<536> Thomas, J. L. (1989). **Gender and perceptions of grandparenthood.** *Inter-
national Journal of Aging and Human Development, 29,* 269-282.

Determines what gender differences arise in 301 seniors' relationships with a grandchild. Finds some differences in grandparenthood meaning and satisfaction, and these
seem to reflect individual personality development, cultural context, and family experience. Grandfathers report less satisfaction than grandmothers. But, gender is not
related to perceived responsibilities, nor the extent to which the grandparent stresses
the centrality of the relationship in their own lives. An earlier finding that grandfathers
express greater responsibility for offering advice and taking care of grandchildren is not
confirmed. They placed emphasis upon generational extension of the family and upon
indulging grandchildren. Grandfathers' stress on indulging grandchildren may reflect
men's nurturance and expressivity in later adulthood, and their endorsement of family
extension is consistent with cultural traditions of patrilineal descent. For grandfathers,
grandchildren have both developmental and cultural importance. [2.3, 8.3]

<537> Tinsley, B. J., & Parke, R. D. (1987). **Grandparents as interactive and so-
cial support agents for families with young infants.** *International Journal
of Aging and Human Development, 25,* 259-277.

Discusses how grandparents engage infants is not well understood. For this work, 30
mothers and 30 fathers, and 30 grandmothers and 21 grandfathers of 7 month-old
infants are observed in separate 5-minute play sessions with the infant in the parents'
homes. Results indicate that both grandfathers and grandmothers are interactive and
provide active support. The pattern of similarities in interactive style is both across
generation and gender. There is a high degree of overlap in parent and grandparent
interaction styles, and gender consistencies are found between the men (fathers and
grandfathers) and women (mothers and grandmothers). [8.3]

MARITAL RELATIONS

<538> Anderson, T. B., & McCulloch, B. J. (1993). Conjugal support: Factor structure for older husbands and wives. *Journals of Gerontology: Social Sciences, 48,* S133-S142.

Investigates the factor structure of social support among 298 older marital couples. Principally examines the dimensionality of social support. Support consists of three factors -- instrumental support, emotional support, and confiding. Finds that rather than conjugal support being a dyadic construct, every marriage consists of his and her versions. For the husbands, confiding and emotional support are strongly interdependent, and instrumental support is more weakly correlated with the other two dimensions. Husbands see instrumental support as an implicit part of the marriage contract, which gives husbands taken-for-granted opportunities to help around the house. [7.5, 8.4]

<539> Berardo, F. M., Appel, J., & Berardo, D. H. (1993). Age dissimilar marriages: Review and assessment. *Journal of Aging Studies, 7,* 93-106.

Reviews the literature of age heterogamy in marriage. Consistent findings in the empirical literature on age dissimilar marriages (ADMs) include: older man/younger woman marriages continue as the most prevalent form of ADMs, ADMs increase with age and with remarriages, non-whites have greater probabilities of age heterogamous marriages, ADMs are most prevalent among lower socioeconomic groups, age disparities differently effect the sexes with respect to mortality, and ADMs appear to be more alike than dissimilar. Findings regarding ADMs and marital stability remain contradictory, partly because definitions of ADMs are arbitrary, show wide variation, and pose impediment to definitive conclusions. [8.4]

<540> Brubaker, T. H., & Kinsel, B. I. (1985). Who is responsible for household tasks in long term marriages of the "young-old" elderly? *Lifestyles, 7,* 238-247.

Examines the division of responsibility for twelve selected household tasks in a sample of 18 couples married 50 years or longer. At least one partner was under 75 years of age. Tasks included cooking meals, washing dishes, yardwork, washing clothes, car maintenance, writing letters, family social events, earning money, cleaning house, shopping, house repairs, and family decisions. Finds that the couples basically develop interdependent, gender-differentiated divisions of household tasks, although they share several tasks. There is congruence between what men and women expected and how they actually divide the responsibility for household tasks. [1.4, 8.4]

<541> Ekerdt, D. J., & Vinick, B. H. (1991). Marital complaints in husband-working and husband-retired couples. *Research on Aging, 13,* 364-382.

Compares marital complaints between 92 older couples in which husbands had been retired one year or less, and 125 couples in which husbands remained employed. Results confirm that retirement is not generally disruptive for older couples, but strains may occur in circumstances that remain to be specified, such as role transitions. [2.3, 8.4, 10.2]

<542> Holahan, C. K. (1986). Marital attitudes over 40 years: A longitudinal and cohort analysis. *Journal of Gerontology, 39*, 49-57.

Investigates changes in marital attitudes from both developmental and historical perspectives. Data for the longitudinal analysis are the Terman Study from 1940 to 1981, when the sample reached age 70; data for the cohort comparison are Stanford alumni who were, on average, age 31. From the longitudinal study, men and women becoming more egalitarian in their attitudes, especially in preference for a declining emphasis on husband's dominance in marriage. However, other traditional gender differences are noted--e.g., older men endorsing a double standard of sexual morality. There is striking evidence that the younger men are involved in family life, yet they and the Terman men at age 30 equally endorse the view that men should wear the pants in the family, thus suggesting developmental and cohort change in attitudes. [1.4, 8.4]

<543> Keith, P. M., & Brubaker, T. H. (1979). Male household roles in later life: A look at masculinity and marital relationships. *Family Coordinator, 28*, 497-502.

Examines men's examines their household roles and marital relationships in late life. Most late life men have intact families and adjust to new family and role expectations. They may adjust by devoting more time to family relationships and homemaking tasks, but to make this adjustment successful, men must be willing to deviate from traditional masculine roles. Research indicates that retired men perform more household tasks as well as tend to concentrate on masculine activities such as repair work and gardening. Retired men who perform household tasks adjust better to retirement. [1.4, 8.4]

<544> Keith, P. M., Schafer, R. B., & Wacker, R. (1992-93). Outcomes of equity/inequity among older spouses. *International Journal of Aging and Human Development, 36*, 187-197.

Determines the association between perceptions of global and specific equity/inequity for 82 couples over age 60. Partners indicate whether they or their spouses are getting a better or an equal deal in their marriage. Finds the employment status of husbands is not associated with his or his wife's perceptions of equity, however husbands whose wives are still in the labor force describe greater inequity. Traditional men recognize they are overbenefited, yet both the traditional men and women felt their relationships are fair. [8.4]

<545> Keith, P. M. (1994). A typology of orientations toward household and marital roles of older men and women. In E. Thompson (Ed.), *Older men's lives* (pp. 141-158). Thousand Oaks, CA: Sage Publications.

Extends the investigation of the congruence and incongruence of husbands' and wives' marital life in the family life cycle. Presents a typology of older men's and women's frames of mind about (or orientations toward) their personal involvement in household work and activities as a husband or wife. The typology profiles four types of spouses -- contented, discontented, strained partners, and strained homemakers. Men are more often contented; they report their work around the home is more manageable, appreciated, and interesting. Contented men report less disagreement and inequity and better well-being than discontented men. Concludes that feeling competent and appreciated is more the providence of older men than older women, and these psychological resources could be an advantage to men's well-being. [1.4, 8.4]

<546> Kuhn, D. R., Morhardt, D. J., & Monbrod-Framburg, G. (1993). Late-life marriages, older stepfamilies, and Alzheimer's disease. *Families in Society, 74,* 154-161.

Investigates the developmental tasks of older stepfamilies such as establishing new traditions, developing a marital bond, and mourning losses. Examines conceptually the impact of a dementing illness on adults married in late life and their stepfamilies. Concludes by offering recommendations for social workers and primary caregivers on what anticipated problems are likely when Alzheimer's disease presents in a stepfamily. [1.5, 2.1, 8.4]

<547> Lee, G. R. (1988). Marital satisfaction in later life: The effects of nonmarital roles. *Journal of Marriage and the Family, 50,* 775-783.

Develops a theory based on role overload and strain which predicts that marital satisfaction is higher in the later stages of the life cycle because of diminishing demands of other, nonmarital roles. Finds very little support for the hypothesis, in fact the findings are contradictory. Rather than distracting husbands from their spouses, involvement in nonmarital roles, including friendships, relations with grandchildren, and church attendance, solidifies older men's marital relationship by integrating the couple. [2.3, 8.4]

<548> Lee, G. R., & Shehan, C. L. (1989). Retirement and marital satisfaction. *Journals of Gerontology: Social Sciences, 44,* S226-S230.

Hypothesizes that both own and spouse's retirement positively affect marital satisfaction, because retirement reduces role conflict and overload and increases time together. Examines the effects of retirement status, length of retirement and spouse's retirement status on marital satisfaction. The hypothesized effects on the quality of marriage are not found for either husbands or wives. Instead, some negative effects are observed, particularly involving effects of husbands' retirement on the marital satisfaction of employed wives. Interpreting the results in terms of equity theory, the authors propose the importance the household division of labor on older husbands' marital satisfaction. [8.4, 10.2]

<549> Levenson, R. W., Carstensen, L. L., & Gottman, J. M. (1993). Long-term marriage: Age, gender, and satisfaction. *Psychology and Aging, 8,* 301-313.

Studies long-term marriages (N = 156) which vary for spouses' age and relative marital satisfaction. Husbands and wives independently complete questionnaires and participate in a laboratory study focused on areas of conflict and sources of pleasure. Husbands report fewer signs of distress, however the relationships between health and marital satisfaction are stronger for wives. Finds support a positive view of older couples' marriages, who evidence reduced potential for conflict, greater potential for pleasure, and less gender differences in sources of pleasure than middle-aged couples. [2.3, 8.4]

<550> Peterson, C. C. (1990). **Husbands' and wives perceptions of marital fairness across the family life cycle.** *International Journal of Aging and Human Development, 31,* 179-188.

Marital fairness, or the subjective balance between two spouses' gains and losses, is evaluated in a sample of 134 married couples representing five points in the family life cycle--preparental, childbearing, the full house, launching, and the postparental empty nest (N = 17). Husbands perceptions of their own marital equity outlines a U-shaped pattern, with more men feeling equitably treated both initially and after children's departure. Wives' perceptions shows little variation. Both sexes tend to agree that whenever deviations from marital equity arose during family life, these are most likely to overbenefit husbands. [8.4]

<551> Szinovacz, M., & Harpster, P. (1993). **Employment status, gender role attitudes, and marital dependency in later life.** *Journal of Marriage and the Family, 55,* 927-940.

Explores perceptions of marital dependence in later life marriages, how couples' employment/retirement patterns affect perceptions of dependence, and whether these relationships are contingent on gender role attitudes. Data are from 673 couples from the National Survey of Families and Households. Husbands' employment-retirement status affects their perceptions of marital dependence in later life marriages, especially if the men endorse more egalitarian gender attitudes. Husbands in dual-retired couples report greater marital dependence than men in dual-earner marriages. Retired men with employed wives do not perceive themselves as dependent on marriage. The findings for husbands are in line with normative resource theory. [8.4, 10.2]

<552> Tucker, M. B., Taylor, R. J., & Mitchell-Kernan, C. (1993). **Marriage and romantic involvement among aged African Americans.** *Journals of Gerontology: Social Sciences, 48,* S123-S132.

Examines the extent and structural correlates of marriage, romantic involvement, and preferences for romantic involvement among older adults in a national sample of 581 African Americans age 55 and older. Analyses indicate that men are more likely than women to be romantically involved and desirous of a romantic involvement, as well as more likely to be married. Age differences are marked: Half of the younger men age 55-64 are romantically involved, but just one in five men age 75 and older are. Forty percent of the 75 and older group desire a romantic involvement (in contrast to 5 percent of the women this age). The authors discuss these patterns in the context of traditional gender role prescriptions and African American men's financial status. [7.4, 8.4]

<553> Uhlenberg, P., & Myers, M. A. P. (1981). **Divorce and the elderly.** *The Gerontologist, 21,* 276-282.

Using Census and vital statistics data, the authors summarize how the 1970s doubling in both the divorce rate and the number of people currently divorce applies equally to elders. Despite this doubling, being divorced in older age is still a relatively uncommon experience, accounting for less than 5 percent of elders. Among elders, divorced older men are noticeable because most older men are married. Divorced men are much less satisfied with their economic position, relations with friends, and family life than all other older, non-married or married men. Greater number of divorced elders are likely because the reduction in mortality, the cohorts entering old age are more accepting of divorce, and women are more economic independent. These divorced elder men are very likely to experience sharp losses in interaction with grandchildren. [2.3, 8.4]

<554> Vinick, B. H., & Ekerdt, D. J. (1991). Retirement: What happens to husband-wife relationships? *Journal of Geriatric Psychiatry*, *24*, 23-40.

Focuses on the effect of husband's retirement on the marriage. Emphasis is on household tasks, companionship activities, personal activities, satisfaction in retirement, and individual-level adjustments and problems. The article concludes that feelings of impingement occur in the first month, but uneasiness lessens as partners develop new routines. [7.4, 8.4, 10.2]

<555> Vinokur, A. D., & Vinokur-Kaplan, D. (1990). In sickness and in health: Patterns of social support and undermining in older married couples. *Journal of Aging and Health*, *2*, 215-241.

Examines the patterns of giving and receiving social support, and the patterns of social undermining (personal criticism) in two samples of older married couples (N = 431). Most wives are either breast cancer survivors or recently diagnosed; some are asymptomatic controls. Husbands report receiving more social support from wives than giving, except in the recently diagnosed group. Advanced age is associated with husbands receiving greater support, and in the two breast cancer groups, of also giving more support and engaging in less undermining. These findings suggests that husband's efforts to provide support are not contingent on the wife's degree of impairment, rather the visibility of diagnosis. [7.5, 8.4, 9.1]

<556> Ward, R. A. (1993). Marital happiness and household equity in later life. *Journal of Marriage and the Family*, *55*, 427-438.

Investigates associations among gender, employment, household task involvement, and marital happiness for 1,355 couples age 50 and older from the National Survey of Families and Households. Gender differences in predictors of fairness and marital happiness are a central interest. Advocacy of egalitarian attitudes for the division of household labor did little in redistribution of household tasks. Men spend fewer hours per week (15) in household tasks than women (37). The older men and women perceive less unfairness to themselves than younger couples, which suggests that older couples hold different expectations. Men may view such tasks as more normative. Perceived unfairness does not affect men's martial happiness, but it does lower women's. [8.4]

<557> Williams, L., & Domingo, L. J. (1993). The social status of elderly women and men within the Filipino family. *Journal of Marriage and the Family*, *55*, 415-426.

Uses cross-sectional data on at least 1,275 adults age 60 and older to assess the relative impact of modernization upon the social status of older men and women in the

Philippines, in particular their decision making power. Although women are apt to control decisions specific to household chores, men have more primary input into the division of labor in the household, participation in community activities, and location of residence. Men's decision making power is reduced by age, exit from the labor force, urban rather than rural residence, and ill-health. [7.1, 8.4]

<558> Wright, L. K. (1991). The impact of Alzheimer's disease on the marital relationship. *The Gerontologist, 31,* 224-237.

Investigates the impact of Alzheimer's disease from a developmental perspective, and examines changes in sexual behavior and marital quality. Afflicted couples (N = 30) are compared with healthy married couples (N = 17). The Alzheimer's couples are incongruent in their perception of tension and agreement over sexual issues. Afflicted spouses perceive much higher marital quality than caregivers. Caregivers differ from well-group spouses on companionship and marital quality. Just one-quarter (27%) of the Alzheimer's couples v. 82% of the well-couples are still sexually active. Of the sexually active, sexual activity was problematic to most of the wife caregivers. [6.2, 8.4, 9.1]

9

Caregiving

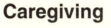

MEN AS CAREGIVERS

<559> Anthony-Bergstone, C. R., Zarit, S. H., & Gatz, M. (1988). Symptoms of psychological distress among caregivers of dementia patients. *Psychology and Aging*, 3, 245-248.

Recognizes a limitation of caregiving research is that most measures of impact have been developed for the caregiving situation specifically. Examines the standardized Brief Symptom Inventory scores of 184 caregivers (including 45 husbands, 51 wives) of dementia patients, and finds all of the caregiving groups are significantly elevated on the hostility subscale. Older wives caring of a husband with dementia appear vulnerable to the stresses of caregiving, and older husbands who are providing care also show elevated symptomatology. [2.3, 9.1]

<560> Arber, S., & Gilbert, G. N. (1989). Transitions in caring: Gender, life course and the care of the elderly. In B. Bytheway, T. Keil, P. Allatt, & A. Bryman (Eds.), *Becoming and being older: Sociological approaches to later life* (pp. 72-92). London: Sage Publications.

Examines why men have been neglected as caregivers and how gender influences the caring trajectory for the elderly-carer relationship. Older men are more likely to take up the responsibilities of the caring role gradually because they have shared a household over a lifetime with the spouse. His "caring for" may be a natural extension of his "caring about," where caring is based on mutual support over a long period of time. Although his caring directly conflicts with masculinity norms as well as the academic paradigm of feminine caring, examining data on the "severely" disabled elders who do not live alone (the General Household Survey for 1980), show elderly husbands and wives are equally likely to be caring for a disabled partner. Concludes that men carers cannot be dismissed. They provide the vast majority of help in relation to bathing and shopping, and the amount of outside help elder husbands receive is not much greater than what elder wives receive. Male carers are less likely to get support and status from their male peers, and may become more isolated from their friendship network. [1.4, 9.1]

<561> Barusch, A. S., & Spaid, W. M. (1989). Gender differences in caregiving: Why do wives report greater burden? *The Gerontologist, 29,* 667-676.

Prior work shows the levels of stress associated with caring for Alzheimer's victims and other frail elders does take a toll. Examines why women typically report greater burden in a sample of 131 caregivers. Among the spouse caregivers, men tend to be older, have more problems with their own health, and perform more caregiving tasks. However, the burden of caregiving is greater among younger wives. Provides four gender-specific explanations for the findings, including men's tendency to be stoic and complain little about caregiving, afflicted husbands are harder to care for than women, and wives experience more negative social contacts with friends, neighbors, and family. [2.3, 2.4, 9.1]

<562> Broden, W., & Berlin, S. (1990). Gender, coping, and psychological well-being in spouses of older adults with chronic dementia. *American Journal of Orthopsychiatry, 60,* 603-610.

Examines 61 spouses caring for their spouse with chronic dementia. Data are from caregivers participating in a larger study on caregiver stress. Results offer little support for the premise of that gender would differentially affect distress and coping. No differences are observed in patients' illness characteristics or distress with symptoms, nor are gender differences noted in reliance on formal support services or the five categories of emotion-focused coping strategies. Gender does emerge as a predictor of psychological well-being; husbands reported lower levels of distress. Queries whether men are expected to demonstrate self-reliance and independence, and approach illness in a more active, instrumental fashion. Older men likely find a sense of purpose in the caregiver role. [2.3, 9.1]

<563> Cicirelli, V. G. (1992). Siblings as caregivers in middle and old age. In J. W. Dwyer, & R. T. Coward (Eds.), *Gender, families, and elder care* (pp. 84-101). Newbury Park, CA: Sage Publications.

Reviews existing literature and describes how gender affects siblings as caregivers of elder family members. Finds sisters provide greater help, and sisters and brothers tend to fulfill tasks depending on how the tasks fit a traditional gender-based division of labor. Concludes that there is not enough evidence to advance the argument that men and women become more androgynous with increasing age, at least in regard to caregiving behavior. Current cohorts of elder siblings appear influenced by gender role stereotypes which override the demands of individual caregiving situations. [8.1, 9.1]

<564> Clipp, E. C., & George, L. K. (1990). Caregiver needs and patterns of social support. *Journals of Gerontology: Social Sciences, 45,* S102-S111.

Predicts four patterns of continuity and change in social support over a one-year interval using levels of caregiver need for 376 adult caregivers of a family member with Alzheimer's disease. Caregiver need does not necessarily elicit support, but need does predict several patterns of support, the most common of which is characterized by high stable support. Older men caregivers have stable low support. [7.5, 9.1]

<565> Cohen, C. A., Gold, D. P., Shulman, K. I., Wortley, J. T., McDonald, G., & Wargon, M. (1993). Factors determining the decision to institutionalize dementing individuals: A prospective study. *The Gerontologist, 33,* 714-720.

Examines longitudinally 196 caregiver/care receiver dyads to determine which variables predict the caregiver decision to institutionalize a dependent with dementia. Determines that although gender did not predict the decision to institutionalize, there is a trend for men to not place their dependents, perhaps because the services used are more effective in helping husbands and because the wives cared for older, frailer dependents. Husbands and wives opt for community care but do not always succeed because of their own age and health. What is predictive are caregivers in poorer health and experiencing greater burden, frail elders' troublesome behavior, and caregiver reactions to that behavior. [2.1, 9.1, 11.2]

<566> Dwyer, J. W., & Seccombe, K. (1991). Elder care as family labor: The influence of gender and family position. *Journal of Family Issues, 12,* 229-247.

Contends that gender differences in caregiving and the amount of time providing care should be reconsidered in the context of family position. Uses a nationally representative sample of noninstitutionalized impaired elders (N = 813) to examine the association of gender and family position with caregiver task performance and total hours of care. Husbands (when compared to wives) and daughters (when compared to sons) spend more time providing care and perform a greater number of caregiving tasks. These findings are controversial and suggest that men and women define caregiving differently and their definitions reflect family position. [9.1]

<567> Enright, R. B. Jr. (1991). Time spend caregiving and help received by spouses and adult children of brain-impaired adults. *The Gerontologist, 31,* 375-383.

Examines how primary caregivers' employment status and kin relationship are associated with amount of help given and the care recipient lives at home or in a care facility. Data are from 155 spouses (55 husbands) and 78 children. Spouse caregivers are much more likely to give care at home and devote larger amounts of time caregiving. Husbands spend no less time than wives. Employed wives and husbands, especially husbands, receive more help from outside sources, particularly paid help. Caregiving wives with the lowest incomes are disadvantaged by traditional gender expectations and receive the least help from family and friends, whereas husbands benefit and receive the most. [7.5, 9.1, 12.3]

<568> Farran, C. J., Keane-Hagerty, E., Salloway, S., Kupferer, S., & Wilken, C. S. (1991). Finding meaning: An alternative paradigm for Alzheimer's disease family caregivers. *The Gerontologist, 31,* 483-480.

Argues that the stress/coping paradigm inadequately explains how persons might grow psychologically and find meaning through their caregiving experiences. Introduces an existential framework to guide the analysis of the experiences of 94 dementia family caregivers (one-third husbands and one-third wives). The analysis reveals that caregivers do express existential themes (e.g., loss and powerlessness, provisional and ultimate meaning), and the search for meaning is primarily an individualized process as opposed to a general process linked to one's race or gender. [9.1]

<569> Fitting, M., Rabins, P., Lucas, M. J., & Eastham, J. (1986). Caregivers for dementia patients: A comparison of husbands and wives. *The Gerontologist, 26,* 248-252.

Maintains that clinicians who work with caregivers believe men and women respond to the caregiver role differently. Compares spouse caregivers of dementia patients on measures of burden, family environment, social networks, psychological adjustment and feelings about the dementing illness. Finds husband and wife caregivers are similar in the perceptions of social environment, experience similar degrees of burden, but wives report more depressive symptoms. When the severity of the dementia increased, some evidence suggests that older husbands and younger wives perceived greater burden. The study fails to affirm the gender difference belief which is prevalent in the developmental literature. [2.3, 7.5, 9.1]

<570> Gallagher, D., Rose, J., Rivera, P., Lovett, S., & Thompson, L. W. (1989). Prevalence of depression in family caregivers. *The Gerontologist, 29,* 444-456.

Seeks to identify the extent of diagnosable clinical depression in several different subgroups of family caregivers. Caregivers who either are seeking help (N = 158) and who volunteer for a longitudinal study of Alzheimer's disease (N = 58) are screened. Among help-seekers, 46 percent met the criteria for depression, while just 18 percent of the non-help-seekers show evidence of a depressive disorder. Older husbands report less dysphoria than wives, and this gender difference is not explained by characteristics of the frail elder or the care the spouse needed. [2.3, 9.1]

<571> Grau, L., Teresi, J. A., & Chandler, B. (1993). Demoralization among sons, daughters, spouses, and other relatives of nursing home residents. *Research on Aging, 15,* 324-345.

Placement of an elder in a nursing home is thought to be a last resort, undertaken only when family members are unable to manage the tasks of caregiving. Finds various aspects of the caregiving situation--caregiver burden, and family members' feelings of guilt and worry about the placement--are related to morale. Analyzing each group of family members separately, spouses are the most vulnerable group, and husbands experience the greatest demoralization. [2.3, 9.1, 11.1]

<572> Gregory, D., Peters, N., & Cameron, C. F. (1990). Elderly male spouses as caregivers--toward an understanding of their experience. *Journal of Gerontological Nursing, 16,* 20-24.

Summarizes how male caregivers have difficulty taking on the personal and household responsibilities and reviews how they cope by focusing on the caregiving tasks and projects, by establishing daily routines, and by carving out their own territory in the home. Husbands as caregivers are more likely than wives to seek the help of formal providers, receive more informal support, but not participate in support groups. Advises nurses to deter\mine elderly husbands' interpretation of caregiving, thereby enabling practitioners to provide support in those areas where burden or difficulties are experienced. [9.1, 12.2]

<573> Harper, S., & Lund, D. A. (1990). **Wives, husbands, and daughters caring for institutionalized and noninstitutionalized dementia patients: Toward a model of caregiver burden.** *International Journal of Aging and Human Development, 30,* 241-262.

Central to the analysis of caregiving burden is the caregiver's gender, relationship to the patient, and the residential location of the patient (same house, community, or institution). Data from 409 caregivers show the primary correlates of burden are the levels and types of elder impairment, and caregiver life satisfaction and social support. Men are less burdened with symptoms of affect; e.g., husbands appear more capable of coping with aggression in their wives than wives are with a violent husband. Husbands have difficulty with the patient's deficits in orientation, particularly when coresidents and others see symptoms of decline in their wives. [9.1, 11.1, 11.2]

<574> Harris, P. B. (1993). **The misunderstood caregiver? A qualitative study of the male caregiver of Alzheimer's disease victims.** *The Gerontologist, 33,* 551-556.

Develops the argument that men in family roles act out of an ethic of duty, and thus men who are caregivers would have less a sense of emotional attachment or commitment to their role as caregivers. In-depth interviews with 15 male caregivers from diverse backgrounds caring for their wives with Alzheimer's disease, finds the following five dominant features and themes: A strong commitment to caregiving, feelings of social isolation from family and friends and the loss of companionship with a wife, coping strategies such as taking control of wives' caregiving and use of respite care, burden lessening and satisfaction rising with years of caregiving, and a need to talk to other men in similar situations. Presents a typology of men who are caregivers: the worker, the labor of love, the sense of duty, and men at the crossroads who were often new caregivers and in crisis. [8.4, 9.1]

<575> Hinrichsen, G. A. (1991). **Adjustment of caregivers to depressed older adults.** *Psychology and Aging, 6,* 631-639.

Interviews older adults hospitalized for major depression and their family caregivers. The primary purpose of the study is to predict caregiver adjustment from caregiver background characteristics, patient illness characteristics, caregiver coping, and strategies for managing the patient at home. Finds better adjustment is associated with the caregiver being in functional health, being male, and being a spouse. Husband caregivers evidence a pattern of adaptation different from daughter, son, and wife caregivers, and concludes that husband caregivers are more emotionally detached from caregiving circumstances and less affected. [2.3, 9.1]

<576> Hooker, K., Frazier, L. D., & Monahan, D. J. (1994). **Personality and coping among caregivers of spouses with dementia.** *The Gerontologist, 34,* 386-392.

Examines the personality and coping strategies among a sample of 50 spouse caregivers of a husband or wife with Alzheimer's disease or a related dementia. Finds through a series of regression analyses that two of the "big five" personality traits explain 60 percent of the variance in emotion-focused coping, 30 percent in problem-focused coping, and 15 percent in social support coping. Gender explains 1, 2, and 5 percent respectively.   Husbands are more likely to use the first two strategies. Concludes that personality is related to coping strategies in caregiving situations much more than gender. [1.3, 9.1]

<577> Kaye, L. W., & Applegate, J. S. (1990). *Men as caregivers to the elderly: Understanding and aiding unrecognized family support.* Lexington, MA: Lexington Books.

Discusses how women traditionally shouldered the responsibility of caring for their frail, elderly relatives. Now, however, as more men enter late life, more older men are taking up the responsibilities of the primary caregiver. Until now, few studies disclose the lives and experiences of men who commit substantial time and energy to caring for elderly members of their families. This seminal work presents the findings from a sample of men caregivers, and provides an in-depth portrait of these men. [1.1,1.4, 9.1]

<578> Kaye, L. W., & Applegate, J. S. (1990). **Men as elder caregivers: A response to changing families.** *American Journal of Orthopsychiatry, 60,* 86-95.

Reports on a study of 148 men who are caregivers, specifically the relationship between their gender orientation and their caregiving experience. The men ascribe to themselves many affective traits. This affective self-definition is correlated with lower caregiving burden, higher frequency of initiating affection, increased levels of affiliation, and a greater sense of competence in caregiving. The majority of the men appear to operate from an ethic of caring. [1.1, 9.1]

<579> Kaye, L. W., & Applegate, J. S. (1994). **Older men and the family caregiving orientation.** In E. Thompson (Ed.), *Older men's lives* (pp. 197-217). Thousand Oaks, CA: Sage Publications.

Recognizes as a distinct minority the older husbands who are involved to a significant degree as a caregiver, and reports research that profiles the characteristics of these caring, older men and their "other-oriented" nurturant orientation. Data are from a sample of 178 white, middle-class men, with the majority older than 60. The men describe themselves as more affective than instrumental, and older husbands in particular do not restrict their range of helping tasks nor ask for outside assistance. Engaged in personal and intense caregiving, their concern is promoting the well-being of dependent family members. They experience distress but remain deeply committed. Predicts that older men's presence among caregivers will swell and advises need to delve deeper into men's experiences. [1.1, 1.4, 9.1]

<580> Lee, G. R. (1993). Gender differences in family caregiving: A fact in search of a theory. In J. W. Dwyer, & R. T. Coward (Eds.), *Gender, families, and elder care* (pp. 120-131). Newbury Park, CA: Sage Publications.

Husbands tend to marry younger wives and women outlive men. This means husbands are likely to need care earlier in the marital life cycle than are wives, and by the time wives need assistance, husbands are often deceased. When adult children provide care, gender is necessary to understand caregiving. The differential roles of sons and daughters in caregiving are specific manifestations of differences in domestic labor, nurturance, and kinship relations. Were these gender-defined domains to change, adult children's patterns of caregiving would change too. [9.1]

<581> Miller, B. (1987). Gender and control among spouses of the cognitively impaired: A research note. *The Gerontologist, 27*, 447-453.

Explores perceptions of caregiving in interviews of 15 elderly spouses caring for a cognitively impaired spouse. Husbands and wives differ in the way they perceive dimensions of control, as observed in their interpretation of the disease process, assumption of authority, control over the environment, and use of social support. These findings suggest a high reliance on previous patterns of gender-role behavior. Men focused on authority and taking charge, whereas the women stressed nurturance and the relationship. [1.3, 8.4, 9.1]

<582> Miller, B., & Cafasso, L. (1992). Gender differences in caregiving: Fact or artifact? *The Gerontologist, 32*, 498-507.

Applies meta-analysis techniques to the results of 14 descriptive studies of gender differences in caregiving, and determines the size and significant of the effects of gender in experience of caregiving stressors and burden. There are essentially no significant gender differences in functional impairment of the frail elder. Nor are there differences in total caregiver involvement or in money management tasks. These similarities support the social role premise that caregivers respond to the demands of the situation. Female caregivers are more likely to carry out personal care and household task, and report greater burden, as predicted by gender socialization. Because the size of the gender effect is small, no consistent paradigm for interpretation of gender and caregiving emerges. [1.1, 9.1]

<583> Miller, B., McFall, S., & Montgomery, A. (1991). The impact of elder health, caregiver involvement, and global stress on two dimensions of caregiver burden. *Journals of Gerontology: Social Sciences, 46*, S9-S19.

Examines the simultaneous effects of an elder's health, caregiver involvement, and stress on caregiver burden with data from the 1982 National Long Term Care Survey. The effect of a frail elder's health and function on personal and interpersonal burden is mediated by task involvement and perceived stress. Contrary to expectation, gender does not have any effect on task involvement. Men who are caregiving report less stress and burden. Attributes associated with gender role and gender socialization may be more important than attributes of the caregiving situation. [2.3, 9.1]

<584> Miller, B., & Montgomery, A. (1990). Family caregivers and limitations in social activities. _Research on Aging, 12,_ 72-93.

Constriction of social and personal activities is one of the most frequently noted consequences among caregivers for frail elders. Using the 1982 National Long Term Care Survey, finds the perceived limitations in social activities vary by gender. Half of the wives and one-third of the husbands who caregive report social limitations. Objective time and energy demands of caregiving are not predictors of who feels constricted; it is the caregiver's subjective appraisal of the nature of providing care. Finds a poor predictive model for husbands and suggests, since caregiving is typically identified as a nurturant role, gender factors may condition men's reaction and adaptation. [7.1, 9.1]

<585> Moritz, D. J., Kasl, S. V., & Ostfeld, A. M. (1992). The health impact of living with a cognitively impaired elderly spouse. _Journal of Aging and Health, 4,_ 244-267.

Identifies the health consequences of living with a cognitively impaired spouse. Data are on 318 couples drawn from a representative sample of noninstitutionalized elderly. Cognitive impairment in wives is significantly associated with elevated systolic blood pressure and perceived declines in health status in husbands. Effects persist after adjusting for influence of wives' functional limitations in activities of daily living and health status, and the perceived adequacy of emotional and instrument support. Concludes health consequences of living with cognitively impaired spouse are great for husbands. [2.2, 9.1]

<586> Motenko, A. K. (1988). Respite care and pride in caregiving: The experience of six older men caring for their disabled wives. In S. Reinharz and G. D. Rowles (Eds.), _Qualitative gerontology_ (pp. 104-127). New York: Springer-Verlag.

Details the subjective meaning of caregiving and respite care to older men. Interviews six white, working-class, retired men age 61 to 88 who are caring for wives with substantial impairments. These men take pride in caregiving and view it as repayment for care their wives had previously given to others. They consider themselves the primary caregivers of their wives, taking responsibility for both their wives' personal care and housekeeping tasks. Caregiving is not associated with stress, rather it allows the husbands to express their love and appreciation. They do not relinquish this responsibility to adult children or professionals, even when assistance is available. They use respite care primarily for rest, errands, or personal activities. Respite care that helps husbands maintain their wives at home contributes to the psychological and physical well-being of both spouses. [8.4, 9.1, 12.3]

<587> Mui, A. C., & Morrow-Howell, N. (1993). Sources of emotional strain among the oldest caregivers: Differential experiences of siblings and spouses. _Research on Aging, 15,_ 50-69.

Investigates whether the strains differ between siblings and spouses, and what sources of role strain apply to both groups. Both groups represent intragenerational family supports of frail elders. The National Long-Term Care Surveys of 1982-1984 have data on 437 spouses and 128 siblings. Finds a high prevalence of role strain among both sibling and spouse caregivers. Role strain is influence by lack of respite support and perceived conflict in personal and social life, especially for siblings. Gender does not emerge as a predictor for role strain among either siblings or spouses. [2.3, 8.1, 9.1]

<588> Pruchno, R. A., & Resch, N. L. (1989). Husbands and wives as caregivers: Antecedents of depression and burden. *The Gerontologist, 29,* 159-165.

Compares the mental health of husband and wife caregivers. Some theorists (e.g., Gutmann) propose that the demands of caregiving is more in line with older men's emerging nurturant tendencies; other theory (e.g., Finch & Groves) suggests that men's socialization makes the demands of caregiving foreign and men less invested in the relationship. This study finds caregiving husbands less depressed than wives, however gender is not a predictor of mental health. There are no predictors of burden for the husbands. Consistent with socialization theory, men are more likely to receive help with the hands-on care; however, inconsistent with this perspective, husbands are more highly invested in the marital relationship than wives. [2.3, 9.1]

<589> Pruchno, R. A., Michaels, J. E., & Potashnik, S. L. (1990). Predictors of institutionalization among Alzheimer disease victims with caregiving spouses. *Journals of Gerontology: Social Sciences, 45,* S259-S266.

Examines a spouse's desire to institutionalize and actual institutionalization within a sample of 220 husbands and wives caring for their spouse with Alzheimer's. There is no simple formula to identify which caregivers place their spouse, and husbands and wives did not differ in propensity. Length of time spent as a caregiver increased likelihood of community residence. The best predictor of placement is the baseline measure of the desire to institutionalize, which seems to be a product of years of consideration and not taken lightly. Other predictors include the greater the number of children and community services used. [9.1, 11.2]

<590> Semple, S. J. (1992). Conflict in Alzheimer's caregiving families: Its dimensions and consequences. *The Gerontologist, 32,* 648-655.

Three conceptually distinct dimensions of family conflict are described and examined in relation to depression and anger. Distinct effects of gender are considered. Self-concepts and normative expectations are implicated as key explanatory variables. [7.5, 9.1]

<591> Stoller, E. P. (1990). Males as helpers: The role of sons, relatives, and friends. *The Gerontologist, 30,* 228-235.

Recognizes men are involved in elder caregiving, and most male caregivers are husbands of the care recipient. This study examines the caregiving contributions of men other than husbands, using interviews with the caregiver and the frail elder at two points in time. Men who are caregivers and not the spouse provide intermittent or occasional assistance and less frequently undertake routine household responsibilities. Helping patterns appear to reflect the cultural division of domestic labor, where men more likely to assist in shopping, financial management, and heavy chores and less likely to assist in daily housekeeping. Evidence that men drop out of caregiving roles when needs intensify is relatively weak, rather the recruit added help and particularly women helpers where the elder's needs escalate to personal care. [9.1]

<592> Stoller, E. P. (1992). **Gender differences in the experiences of caregiving spouses.** In J. W. Dwyer, & R. T. Coward (Eds.), *Gender, families, and elder care* (pp. 49-64). Newbury Park, CA: Sage Publications.

Uses the available literature to address the experiences of husbands and wives caring for disabled partners. Discusses how the gender of the spouse caregiver has a significant effect on the meaning and consequences of the caregiving role. For example, husbands and wives seem to have different tolerance thresholds, with men less burdened but more likely to institutionalize. Husbands focus on caregiving tasks and extend their instrumental role to this context, while wives are more likely to empathize and experience their husband's disability. The chapter calls attention to the dearth of information on less advantaged couples, non-white couples, and the effects of marital history. [8.4, 9.1]

<593> Stoller, E. P., & Cutler, S. J. (1992). **The impact of gender on configurations of care among married elder couples.** *Research on Aging, 14,* 313-330.

Understands spouse caregivers are the first line of assistance in providing care to a disabled elder, and husbands and wives bring different experiences and resources to the role of caregiver. Analyzes data from the Supplement on Aging to the 1984 National Health Interview Schedule for gender differences in the configuration of care among married elder couples. Most spouses (greater than 80 percent) do not have any difficulties with activities in daily living, and nine of ten married couples who experience some ADL difficulty manage on their own. Husband caregivers are likely to incorporate extra-household assistance, but they are no more likely to incorporate paid help than they are to rely on informal sources. The results are consistent with several explanations available in the literature; four are outlined. [9.1, 12.3]

<594> Stone, R., Cafferata, G. L., & Sangl, J. (1987). **Caregivers of the frail elderly: A national profile.** *The Gerontologist, 27,* 616-626.

The 1982 National Long-Term Care Survey and Informal Caregivers Survey provide data for the first national estimates of informal caregivers to noninstitutionalized disabled elders. This article provides a descriptive profile. Affirming prior work, informal caregivers are primarily spouses and daughters. Husbands, typically overlooked in the caregiver research, are the oldest subgroup of caregivers, and they reported spending the greatest number of extra hours fulfilling caregiving responsibilities. Half provide this care with no informal or paid assistance. Two-thirds of the wives caring for frail their husbands are 65 or older, and nearly half of these wives define their own health as fair or poor. The authors encourage research on spouse caregivers. [9.1]

<595> Tennstedt, S. L., Crawford, S., & McKinlay, J. B. (1993). **Determining the pattern of community care: Is coresidence more important than caregiver relationship.** *Journals of Gerontology: Social Sciences, 48,* S74-S83.

It is argued that spouses are a distinct group of caregivers--they provide more care with less help from others. However, based on the theory of primary groups, this study hypothesizes that coresidence is more important than kinship in determining the pattern of caregiving. When spouses are compared to other coresiding caregivers, patterns of informal care and use of formal services are similar. Elder husband caregivers do spent greater amounts of time in housekeeping tasks, which is attributed to men's new housekeeping activities and prior lack of experience. Elder men who receive assistance have a high rate of assistance with meals. Variance in amounts of care provided and received is explained best by coresidence, gender and frailty level, not the caregiver relationship. [9.1, 11.2, 12.3]

<596> Tennstedt, S. L., McKinlay, J. B., & Sullivan, L. M. (1989). Informal care for frail elders: The role of secondary caregivers. *The Gerontologist*, 29, 677-683.

Most studies of informal care examine only the role and activities of the primary caregiver, but most elders (nearly three-quarters) receive help from other caregivers as well. This study describes the identity and activities of these secondary caregivers, who are half of the time the children and in-laws of the elder, or the spouse or children of the primary caregiver. Men (particularly sons-in-law) are more likely a secondary caregiver than a primary one, and on average, these secondary men provide more care (13 hours weekly) than secondary women. As supplementary caregivers, they are involved less in personal care and more in intermittent help.   [9.1, 9.2]

<597> Vitaliano, P. P., Russo, J., Young, H. M., Teri, L., & Maiuro, R. D. (1991). Predictors of burden in spouse caregivers of individuals with Alzheimer's disease. *Psychology and Aging*, 6, 392-402.

Presents longitudinal data to evaluate a dynamic model of distress (or burden) among husbands and wives providing care for spouses with Alzheimer's. Algebraically, distress is a function of exposure to stressors plus vulnerability divided by psychological and social resources. Level of distress at onset is significantly related to gender, with husbands more distressed with caregiving. Long-term burden, however, is no longer correlated with gender. [2.3, 9.1]

<598> Williamson, G. M., & Schulz, R. (1990). Relationship orientation, quality of prior relationship, and distress among caregivers of Alzheimer's patients. *Psychology and Aging*, 5, 502-509.

Investigates communal orientation and closeness of relationship as predictors of caregivers' distress. Persons high in communal orientation are less depressed, and caregivers who report a close relationship with the patient before illness onset fell less burdened. However, communal orientation and closeness interact when data are analyzed for men and women separately. Among men, being low in communal orienta-tion and having a relatively poor prior relationship are associated with the highest levels of depression, levels that put them at risk for clinical depression. Perhaps, these men are distressed about by the cultural expectations to provide a high level of help to someone with whom their past experiences have not been rewarding. [2.3, 9.1]

<599> Young, R. F., & Kahana, E. (1989). Specifying caregiver outcomes: Gender and relationship aspects of caregiving strain. *The Gerontologist, 29,* 660-666.

In a study of 183 heart patient-caregiver dyads, analyzes the importance of gender and relationship singly and jointly for both the process and outcome of caregiving. Data are collected six weeks and one year after hospital discharge. There are consistent patterns of strain. Husbands averaged 22 hours of weekly care, wives 35 hours, and daughters 32; yet, this difference is not greater than chance. Task-specific findings show that wives prepare meals more than others, husbands do laundry as much as wives, the handiwork needs, and (along with daughters) assist with transportation. Husbands report the least burden, mental distress, role conflict, and physical health decline; and, husband and wife caregivers differ significantly from each other.   [2.3, 9.1]

<600> Zarit, S. H., Todd, P. A., & Zarit, J. M. (1986). Subjective burden of husbands and wives as caregivers: A longitudinal study. *The Gerontologist, 26,* 260-266.

A two-year follow-up of a sample of husband and wife caregivers of spouses with dementia is conducted to determine decision to institutionalize and changes over time for caregiver feelings. Caregivers' ability to tolerate problem behaviors actually increases, even as the disease progresses. Nursing home placement is more strongly associated with subjective factors, particularly caregivers' perceived burden, than it is with objective indicators such as the severity of dementia. The difference in subjective burden reported by husbands and wives at time 1 are no longer apparent in the two-year follow-up, possibly because wives adopt the more instrumental coping style typical of men. [2.3, 9.1, 11.2]

FAMILY DEPENDENCIES

<601> Cattanach, L., & Tebes, J. K. (1991). The nature of elder impairment and its impact on family caregiver's health and social functioning. *The Gerontologist, 31,* 246-255.

Examines the effect of elder impairment on the health and well-being of the daughters and daughters-in-law who live in the same household. Contrary to previous research, finds no self-reported health and well-being differences across caregivers of cognitively impaired, functionally impaired, and nonimpaired elderly relatives. Nor does the elder's gender or, most times, the cross-sex relationship affect caregivers' health and well-being. Concludes that caregiver gender, living arrangement, and the caregiving context (family generation) affect the caregiver more than the elder's characteristics. [2.3, 2.4, 9.2]

<602> Coward, R. T., Horne, C., & Dwyer, J. W. (1992). Demographic perspectives on gender and family caregiving. In J. W. Dwyer, & R. T. Coward (Eds.), *Gender, families, and elder care* (pp. 18-33). Newbury Park, CA: Sage Publications.

Observes that older men appear highly dependent on their wives as sources of assistance.   Finds two-thirds of the frail older men report receiving help from wives, compared to one in five older women receiving help from husbands. Fewer older men report receipt of help from adult children, but when they do, sons are nearly as present as daughters in older men's helping networks. These patterns differ as men age, with children and hired help replacing wives. [9.2]

<603> Himes, C. L. (1992). Future caregivers: Projected family structures of older persons. *Journals of Gerontology: Social Sciences, 47*, S17-S26.

Reviews how elders depend upon spouses and children for emotional, physical, and financial support, and estimates the demographic determinants of family status and family caregivers for 2020. The projections separate the elder population by sex and race into status groups which are based on the presence of spouses and children. Changes in past and future levels of fertility, marriage, divorce and mortality suggest that elderly persons in the near future will have surviving spouses and children. Declines in mortality, coupled with increases in rates of marriage, increase the probability that both men and women will have spouses surviving in their old age. [9.2]

<604> Koch, T. (1990). *Mirrored lives: Aging children and elderly parents.* New York: Praeger.

Chronicles as a narrative record the caregiving relationship a son (the author) constructs for his elderly father. The older man live is transformed from one of independence and social and financial worth to one of being a geriatric parent and patient who experiences decreased mobility, increasing senility, and the ill-effects of psychological distress. [9.2]

<605> Miller, B., & McFall, S. (1991). The effect of caregiver's burden on change in frail older persons' use of formal helpers. *Journal of Health and Social Behavior, 32*, 165-179.

Assesses the probabilities of the transition to using formal helpers within the two-year period. Uses a national longitudinal sample of elders (N = 940) and their caregivers to determine the importance of predisposing factors (e.g., elder's age, race, gender), enabling factors (e.g., number of informal caregivers), the level of older person's functional disability and need, and caregiver's sense of burden in utilization of formal helpers. Finds use of formal helpers is greater in situations combining high levels of older person's functional disability and need, high levels of caregiver's personal burden, and insufficient support from the informal network. Neither elder's gender nor the caregiver being a spouse affect requests for formal service providers. [9.2, 12.3]

<606> Miller, B., & McFall, S. (1992). Caregiver burden and the continuum of care: A longitudinal perspective. *Research on Aging, 14*, 376-398.

Examines the effects of caregiver burden over a two-year period and reviews ways in which burden alters the caregiving.   Two dimensions of burden---personal and interpersonal---are constructed from the 1982-1984 National Long Term Care Survey. Neither aspect of burden has an independent effect on changes in the informal task support network, and over the two years continuity of care is high and responsive to changing care needs.   Personal burden does influence the introduction of formal services--home care or nursing home placement. Gender of frail elder does not emerge as a predictor of the elder's institutionalization. [9.2, 11.2]

<607> Montgomery, R. J. V., & Hirshorn, B. A. (1991). Current and future family help with long-term care needs of the elderly. *Research on Aging, 13*, 171-204.

Provides an description of the sociodemographic composition of the older population and its primary kin support. Data from the sample of age 60 and older from the National Survey of Families and Households reveal the probability for men having a spouse or child available to help is greater than for women. Indeed the absence of close kin is one-half as likely for men as for women--10.2% of all men age 60 and over, 13.6% for women. Black males age 60 to 69 have the greatest chance of having a spouse or child potentially available for support. These patterns of kin availability reflect the presence and absence of a coresident spouse. [7.5, 8.4, 9.2]

10

Economics and Retirement

— ◆ —

ECONOMIC WELL-BEING

<608> Burkhauser, R. V., Butler, J. S., & Holden, K. C. (1991). **How the death of a spouse affects economic well-being after retirement: A hazard model approach.** *Social Science Quarterly, 72,* 504-519.

Reveals with cross-sectional data that among elders, widows and widowers are significantly worse off economically than married couples. Traces families of married men who retired during the ten year Retirement History Study, and finds the incidence of a fall into poverty and of a significant drop in the income-to-needs ratio dramatically increases for widows and less so for widowers. Widowers are more likely to experience a bad economic period prior to the death of a spouse than following it. [10.1]

<609> Clark, R. (1992-93). **Modernization and status change among aged men and women.** *International Journal of Aging and Human Development, 36,* 171-186.

Comments how cross-national investigations of modernization support the theory that the status of elders in a community is inversely related to the degree of modernization. Investigates the relationship between elderly occupational status and modernization for men and for women. Finds economic development is associated with the relative losses of elder men in professional and technical occupations, but not administrative or managerial occupations. Development seems to adversely affect elderly women more than elderly men, because modernization benefits younger women. [10.1, 12.1]

<610> Coe, R. D. (1988). **A longitudinal examination of poverty in the elderly years.** *The Gerontologist, 28,* 540-544.

Studies the relationships among gender, increasing age, and poverty in later life. Using the Panel Study of Income Dynamics, finds a conspicuous gender-based distinction in the experience of poverty. Elderly men have a considerably higher probability of escaping poverty than elderly women. During the first three years of poverty, men's exit probabilities were relatively high, much like the probabilities in the non-elderly years.

However, after spending three elderly years in poverty, the probability of escaping poverty is extremely low. [10.1]

<611> Covey, H. C. (1991). Old age and historical examples of the miser. *The Gerontologist, 31,* 673-678.

Notes how social constructions of older people have historically characterized them as avaricious and miserly. Reviews historical reasons for characterizing older people as misers, such as their need to control wealth, intergenerational conflict, and lack of social support programs. The "miser" is linked to the role of "paterfamilias" and to old men, because of the association of men with wealth and because of the stereotype of father resented by his children. Concludes that in modern times, there is a decline in use of these constructed images. [6.2, 10.1, 12.1]

<612> Crystal, S., Shea, D., & Krishnaswami, S. (1992). Educational attainment, occupational history, and stratification: Determinants of later-life economic outcomes. *Journals of Gerontology: Social Sciences, 47,* S213-S221.

Investigates the determinants of economic well-being among men age 25-44, 45-64, and 65 and older using the 1984 panel of the Survey of Income and Program Participation. This study explores the effects of education, race, and occupational history on men's "wealth," adjusted for assets, household composition, and underreporting of unearned income. Finds education effects are undiminished as men become elders; education explains more of the variance in adjusted income for the elderly than the nonelderly. Income is derived mainly from benefits and assets. The nonelderly's income is dominated by earnings. Social Security has no an equalizing effect across educational attainment groups, yet private pensions and other important retirement income sources are highly education-dependent. [10.1]

<613> Elder, G. H., Pavalko, E. K., & Hastings, T. J. (1991). Talent, history, and the fulfillment of promise. *Psychiatry, 54,* 251-267.

Explores the long-term consequences of an era of social change--World War II and the preceding decade of economic depression--for the life experiences and career achievements of men who lived through that period. Using data archives from Terman's (1925) longitudinal study, the career achievements of men born 1904-1917 are assessed in relation to cohort membership, social origins, and wartime mobilization. Finds the life stages of these men in the 1930s and 1940s provided different opportunities, recourses, and support and, thus, differentially shaped the distinctive impact of the historical circumstances on their own accomplishments. [1.4, 4.4, 10.1]

<614> Fillenbaum, G. G., George, L. K., & Palmore, E. B. (1985). Determinants and consequences of retirement among men of different races and economic levels. *Journal of Gerontology, 40,* 85-94.

Draws on two national longitudinal studies (Longitudinal Retirement History Survey, National Longitudinal Survey) of older workers to compare the determinants and consequences of retirement for white and black men whose economic level is one of poverty, marginally above poverty, or an upper level. The number of determinants affecting retirement is greater for white men than for black men, and the number increase with economic level. Retirement has few direct consequences. It is consequential for health and economic matters. Men at the marginal economic level are affected most adversely. Blacks and poverty level men are minimally affected by retirement, perhaps because the impact of retirement is somewhat ameliorated by age-determined income maintenance programs and subsidies. [10.1]

<615> Ginn, J., & Arber, S. (1991). Gender, class and income inequalities in later life. *British Journal of Sociology, 42*, 369-396.

Using the 1985 and 1986 General Household Survey (United Kingdom) on a sample of over 7000 people age 65 and older, focuses on the gender inequality of occupational and private pension income. Discusses the effects of the division in labor market by gender and the "advantages" of being male. Concludes that gender and marital status (being married) are crucial factors determining income inequality among elders. [10.1]

<616> Gohmann, S. F. (1990). Retirement differences among the respondents to the Retirement History Survey. *Journals of Gerontology: Social Sciences, 45*, S120-S127.

Raises as an empirical question whether the Social Security reforms encourage paid work in later life equally for white and black men who also differ in marital status. Studies have simulated the effect of changes in the Social Security system on the retirement age of married white men. The retirement decisions of single people, blacks, and women, however, seem to differ. Because black men and women and single white women have substantially lower retirement wealth and Social Security makes up a larger portion of their total wealth, their retirement decisions do not compare to married white men. Concludes that variation among older men must be taken into account-- single white men and single black men are not well represented by these research examining retirement responses of married white men. [10.1, 12.3]

<617> Gustman, A. L., & Steinmeier, T. L. (1986). A disaggregated, structural analysis of retirement by race, difficulty of work and health. *Review of Economics and Statistics, 68*, 509-513.

Analyzes the retirement probabilities separately for blacks and whites in the Retirement History Survey. Using structural retirement models to analyze men's responsiveness to retirement, observes that the very wide black-white differentials in rates of full time employment participation typically found for middle aged men decline with age. Concludes that the "responsiveness" of men in poor health and in difficult, physically demanding jobs to the work incentives in the 1983 Social Security Amendments will be sufficient to, on average, increase these groups' earnings. [10.1, 10.2]

<618> Hanks, R. S. (1990). The impact of early retirement incentives on retirees and their families. *Journal of Family Issues, 11*, 424-437.

Uncertainty was introduced with the widespread use of incentive-based early retirement as a work force reduction strategy during the 1980's. Explores 60 men's and (when available) their wives' perceptions of early retirement on themselves and their families. Retirees are satisfied with early retirement, and satisfaction is significantly related to health and expectations for the future health and productivity. By comparison, spouses are generally satisfied but expressed concerns about the husband's adjustment and their own loss of privacy. [10.1, 10.2]

<619> Hardy, M. A., & Hazelrigg, L. E. (1993). The gender of poverty in an aging population. *Research on Aging, 15*, 243-278.

Addresses the increasing feminization of poverty, especially among elderly households. Using data from a 1986 survey of Florida's resident population age 55 and over, analyzes the gender differential in correlates of poverty--race/ethnicity, education, income sources, and living arrangement. Men experience little or no decline in relative economic resource after spousal death; some evidence suggest that widowers' economic circumstances are likely to improve, not worsen. By comparison, many women spend the bulk of their adult lives as financial dependents in a martial relationship or as working unmarried women in an economic culture that viewed women's employment as irrelevant to a family's financial security. Once their spouses precede them in death, women, not men, shift from one status of economic dependence to another. [10.1]

<620> Hayward, M. D., Grady, W. R., & McLaughlin, S. (1988). Changes in the retirement process among older men in the United States: 1972-1980. *Demography, 25*, 371-386.

Changes in Social Security benefits, the mandatory retirement age, life expectancy, and the economy in the 1970s compel a re-examination of older men's retirement patterns, particularly whether or not changes in the retirement transition is homogeneous across occupations. Finds labor force incumbents are unequally "sheltered" from policy and economic changes. Those in secondary occupations are less sheltered from macrolevel changes. Although working life expectancy remains relatively stable across occupations, men in secondary occupations spent increasingly greater portions of their work lives in postretirement jobs. The large increases in nonworking-life expectancy occur more because of general increases in life expectancy than declines in working-life expectancy. [10.1, 10.2]

<621> Hayward, M. D., & Grady, W. R. (1990). Work and retirement among a cohort of older men in the United States. *Demography, 27*, 337-356.

Recognizes that one in three men return to the labor force after retirement. The flood of older men reentering the labor force is a direct result of declines in the age of first retirement. Former blue-collar workers are more likely to come out of retirement for financial reasons, but former professionals are more likely to go back to work because they enjoy it. Marked differences in labor force mobility and in working and nonworking life expectancy vary according to occupation, class of worker, education, race, and marital status. Discusses the implications of these findings for inequities of access to retirement, private and public pension consumption, and future changes in the retirement process. [10.1, 10.2]

<622> Hayward, M. D., & Liu, M. C. (1992). **Men and women in their retirement years: A demographic profile.** In M. Szinovacz, D. J. Ekerdt, & B. H. Vinick (Eds.), *Families and retirement* (pp. 23-50). Newbury Park, CA: Sage Publications.

Provides a demographic overview of the work and familial situations of older Americans who are near the age of retirement. Analyses are based on data on 5,259 men and 6,302 women from the Survey of Income and Program Participation by the U. S. Bureau of the Census. The authors observe substantial effects of birth cohort in shaping much of the age heterogeneity among older men -- such as variations in education, participation in military service, and employed wives. Emphasizes the need to recognize that the work and family characteristics of elderly men will change much more visibly in the future. Diversity is increasingly important because it signals the variability across subgroups of men (and women) in their capability to maintain a quality of life. [10.1]

<623> Keith, P. M. (1985). **Financial well-being of older divorced/separated men and women: Findings from a panel study.** *Journal of Divorce, 9,* 61-72.

Compares the objective and subjective financial well-being of older divorced/separated men (N = 114) and women (N = 251) at the beginning and end of a 10-year period. Data are from the 1969 and 1979 panels of the Longitudinal Retirement History Study. Finds men and women do not differ in satisfaction with their level of living or adequacy of income at either assessment. Men's perception of income adequacy is more strongly effected by actual income. Over the ten years, divorce has a negative influence on men's assessments of finances, perhaps reflecting that their earnings fail to increase as much as expected or their costs fail to decrease as much as expected. [10.1]

<624> Keith, P. M., & Lorenz, F. O. (1989). **Financial strain and health of unmarried older people.** *The Gerontologist, 29,* 684-691.

Scrutinizes two life areas in which the 1,782 unmarrieds seem to fare less well than the married -- health and finances. No evidence emerges to demonstrate financial strain aggravates health or contributes to poorer health among unmarrieds. Finds the effect of greater financial strain earlier in life is not related to physical health a decade later, nor is there congruence between objective circumstance (financial hardship) and subjective evaluation (financial strain). Also finds unmarried men are much more dissatisfied with their finances despite being objectively better off than women. Concludes that elders scale down aspirations and do not negatively construct their situation. [2.2, 2.3, 10.1]

<625> Meyer, D. R., & Bartolomei-Hill, S. (1994). **The adequacy of Supplemental Security Income benefits for aged individuals and couples.** *The Gerontologist, 34,* 161-172.

Provides information on the adequacy of benefits using state-level data on costs and benefits. Maximum SSI benefits for aged persons are generally shown to be inadequate, however when income from other sources is included, couples' SSI benefits appear more adequate. Unmarried and formerly married older men's and women's SSI benefits remain inadequate. [10.1, 12.1]

<626> Moen, J. R. (1988). Past and current trends in retirement: American men from 1860-1980. *Economic Review, 73*, 16-27.

The decreasing participation in the labor force of men age 65 and older emerged as a unique phenomenon in the middle of this century. In 1985, 16 percent of older men worked outside the home; by comparison, 58 percent of men in this age bracket were in the labor force in 1930. Three changes between 1860 and 1980 account for the decreased participation: In 1860, most people worked on farms and there was little reason to retire completely. By the late 1930's Social Security and pensions began to be offered to workers by businesses. Younger workers were preferred for assembly line work. The growth of private pension plans and Social Security, as well as rising real income, wages, and unearned income, play a role, however, the trend in lower labor force participation among older men has stopped declining and may even be increasing. [10.1, 10.2]

<627> Mueller, C. W., Mutran, E., & Boyle, E. H. (1989). Age discrimination in earnings in a dual-economy market. *Research on Aging, 11*, 492-507.

Age discrimination in earnings has been difficult to establish because of the confounding effects of human capital variables that deteriorate as workers age. Examines the age-earnings for a panel of older workers in 1966 and 1976. No matter how thorough the measurement of worker background, education, training, experience, job characteristics, and labor market conditions, age-based wage discrimination is found for core (not periphery) sector workers, and as expected, becomes more prevalent as workers grow older. These findings affirm how core employees lose power in the work place, and how older core employees are disadvantaged. [6.1, 10.1]

<628> Piachaud, D. (1986). Disability, retirement and unemployment of older men. *Journal of Social Policy, 15*, 145-162.

Examines changes in the economic position of older men in relation to changing rates of unemployment. Among older men in England from 1971 to 1981, the increase in the extent of those defined as disabled is of the same order as the increase in unemployment. Census data for the forty-six counties of England show changes in disability and retirement are in fact directly related to changes in unemployment. A substantial proportion of the overall increase in disability and the decline in economic activity is attributable to the general rise in unemployment. [10.1, 10.2]

<629> Richardson, V., & Kilty, K. M. (1989). Retirement financial planning among black professionals. *The Gerontologist, 29*, 32-37.

Researchers commonly generalizes to blacks from studies of predominantly white populations. Compares the extent and patterns of financial planning among 234 black professionals with those of white professionals. Finds some similarities--greater income and age remain influential predictors of planning. Unlike whites, black men who do not have dependent children are more likely to have pension resources. Gender is not influential in the analysis of blacks' investments, planning, or proportion of income retained; among whites men and women differ in their use of these three types of resources. Black men and women may differ in their labor force participation, but the differences are minimal and much less than between white men and women. [10.1]

<630> Rones, P. L. (1978). Older men--The choice between work and retirement. *Monthly Labor Review, 101* (11), 3-10.

Reviews how rising retirement income sent rates of participation in the labor force plummeting among older men, from 82 percent of those age 60-64 in 1957 to 63 percent twenty years later. Although some older men work part time for health reasons, others do so to supplement low benefits. The greatest declines in work participation among men occur between 61 and 62 (from 70 to 56 percent) and between 64 to 65 (from 48 to 83 percent). [10.1]

<631> Taylor, R. J., & Chatters, L. M. (1988). Correlates of education, income, and poverty among aged blacks. *The Gerontologist, 28*, 435-441.

Disadvantaged employment and economic conditions among blacks are evident across the life-span. This work examines the demographic correlates of education, income, and poverty in a national sample of elderly black adults (N = 581). These data indicate that gender, marital status, age, employment status, urban residence and region differentially predict. Despite older black men having no greater educational attainment than older black women, they have higher incomes and less poverty. [10.1]

<632> Wolfson, M., Rowe, G., Gentleman, J. F., & Tomiak, M. (1993). Career earnings and death: A longitudinal analysis of older Canadian men. *Journals of Gerontology: Social Sciences, 48*, S167-S179.

Reports an analysis of men's mortality at ages 65 to 74 in relation to socioeconomic characteristics--specifically, their employment and self-employment earning histories the 10-20 years prior to age 65. Data are from the Canada Pension Plan. Finds mortality gradients throughout the earning spectrum. Married men have significantly higher survival probabilities at all retirement ages, and high earnings entail high survival probabilities, but the magnitude of this earnings gradient narrows for later retirement ages. In effect, an extra dollar of income is "beneficial" for longevity at all income levels and at each age, but it offers a decreasing protective effect at higher incomes. [10.1]

<633> Zick, C. D., & Smith, K. R. (1986). Immediate and delayed effects of widowhood on poverty: Patterns from the 1970s. *The Gerontologist, 26*, 669-675.

Research shows a family's economic well-being is more likely to change because of a shift in family composition. This study examines the economic consequences of widowhood for both men and women over time. Compares their financial well-being to that of a matched group of continuously married couples. In a sample of initially nonpoor widowed individuals, the loss of a spouse is associated with dramatic declines in economic well-being for both widows and widowers relative to continuously married couples. Widowers experience economic hardships as dramatic as those endured by widows. [10.1]

WORK/RETIREMENT

<634> Anson, O., Antonovsky, A., Sagy, S., & Adler, I. (1989). Family, gender, and attitudes toward retirement. *Sex Roles, 20*, 355-369.

Examines the relationships among marital status, proximity of children, and attitudes toward retirement for 432 men and 373 women on the verge of retirement. Three types of attitudes were studied -- attitudes toward losses associated with retirement, toward gains in entering retirement, and toward gains in leaving work. Men report more negative attitudes toward both gains; there are no gender differences concerning attitudes toward losses. The married of both sexes perceive more gains with the transition to retirement. [10.2]

<635> Antonovsky, A., & Sagy, S. (1990). Confronting developmental tasks in the retirement transition. *The Gerontologist, 30*, 362-368.

Presents retirement as a widespread developmental transition for individuals, and reconceptualizes the retirement transitions using Erikson's life cycle model. Retirement is viewed as a transition involving phase-specific psychosocial crises, tasks, and challenges (e.g., challenge between generativity and integrity). Draws a distinction between developmental tasks and outcomes, and identifies four central tasks--active involvement, reevaluation of the sources of life satisfaction, reevaluation of one's world view, and attending to a personal sense of health maintenance. [1.4, 10.2]

<636> Beck, S. H. (1982). Adjustment to and satisfaction with retirement. *Journal of Gerontology, 37*, 616-624.

Reports on retirees' psychological well-being (happiness with life). Using the National Longitudinal Surveys of Mature Men, finds the loss of the work role does not have a significant negative effect on personal happiness. However, men retiring much earlier than they expected are less likely to be happy with their lives compared to men still in the labor force. Health and income are important factors in personal happiness as well as in the evaluation of retirement. The experience of divorce, separation, or widowhood predictably has a negative effect on the personal happiness. [2.3, 10.2]

<637> Beck, S. H. (1985). Determinants of labor force activity among retired men. *Research on Aging, 7*, 251-280.

Investigates what effects work activity during retirement. Includes the effects of social and demographic factors, preretirement attitudes toward work, health, and mediating factors such as retirement benefits. Uses the National Longitudinal Surveys, and finds job opportunities which emerge from one's preretirement occupation do affect decision to work, however the individual-level issues of poor health and low retirement benefits are more pivotal in determining labor force activity among retired men. [2.1, 10.2]

<638> Beck, S. H. (1986). Mobility from preretirement to postretirement job. *Sociological Quarterly, 27*, 515-531.

Details the amount of employment and occupational mobility among the "working-retired." Data are from the older men's cohort of the National Longitudinal Surveys. Approximately one-third of the men work during their retirement, and the structure of mobility is found to be similar to younger labor force participants. Most mobility consists of moves to adjacent occupational categories. Unlike career mobility, the majority of moves among the working-retirees constitutes downward mobility. [10.2]

<639> Berkovec, J., & Stern, S. (1991). Job exit behavior of older men. *Economet-rica, 59*, 189-210.

Conceptualizes retirement decisions and job exit behavior for older men as "economic" decisions workers make involving wage and leisure value-based choices. The model is dynamic, for each individual chooses when to make job state changes and which changes to make at any time. The research models reveal that poor health, age, and lack of education increase the probability of retirement. [10.2]

<640> Bikson, T. K., & Goodchilds, J. D. (1991). *Experiencing the retirement transition: Managerial and professional men before and after.* Santa Monica, CA: Rand.

Summaries research examining the social psychological factors involved in the transition to retirement in 179 managerial and professional men. Four areas are addressed: use of time, family and social adjustment, self-construct, and retirement planning process. Retirees are significantly more satisfied than employees with their overall use of time, especially so for time spent with spouse. Those who report a greater proportion of time spent with their wives perceive themselves more as part of a pair and are significantly happier with their marital arrangements than others, regardless of employment status. Retirees make more new friends than employees, in the neighborhood and among colleagues. Retirees' and employees' scores on measures of self-esteem, loneliness, and other psychological constructs are similar, nor do retirees and employees differ in degree of integration into social life. Concludes there is a positive effect of planning adequately for retirement. [10.2]

<641> Blank, A. M., Ritchie, P. J., & Ryback, D. (1983). Lack of satisfaction in post-retirement years. *Psychological Reports, 53*, 1223-1226.

Addresses the difficulty associated with retirement in a sample of 32 retired men who's average age is 69 and who are still participating in paid work. The men had worked full time for at least ten years and are working less than fifteen hours per week. Question-naire responses suggest lack of satisfaction with post-retirement life. [2.3, 10.2]

<642> Boaz, R. F. (1987). Early withdrawal from the labor force: A response only to pension pull or also to labor market push? *Research on Aging, 9*, 530-547.

Observes that not-yet-old men whose health is not failing are retiring from the labor market at a time when they do not receive any pension income and the level of their nonwage income is very low. Examines why these men stop working as early as they do, instead of continuing to work at least until they are old enough to claim Social Se-curity benefits. Early retirement cannot be attributed solely to the pull of pensions. Adverse labor market conditions result in diminished employment opportunities and push older workers out. The latter is more likely for lifetime employees than self-employed men. [10.1, 10.2]

<643> Boaz, R. F., & Muller, C. F. (1989). Does having more time after retirement change the demand for physician services? *Medical Care, 27*, 1-15.

Investigates whether discouraging early retirement, which was the intent of the 1983 Amendments to the Social Security Act, will reduce the use of medical services, on the assumption that persons who continue to work would have less structured time than retirees for physicians. Studies 1,876 men born between 1907 and 1910. Finds retired men do not increase the demand for ambulatory services, compared to being a part-time or full-time employee. Compared to men in full-time self-employment, however, the probability of using any physician services increases in the year by 14 percent and the number of physician visits by two visits. Concludes other factors influence physician visits -- Medicare coverage, private health insurance, income, education, and health status. [10.2, 12.2]

<644> Bosse, R., Aldwin, C. M., Levenson, M. R., & Workman-Daniels, K. (1991). How stressful is retirement? Findings from the Normative Aging Study. *Journals of Gerontology: Psychological Sciences*, *46*, P9-P14.

Investigates the stressfulness of retirement as a life stage and as a transitional event experienced during the past year. Transitional stress is assessed using a life events approach and stage stress uses a "hassles" approach. Data are from the 1,516 men in the Normative Aging Study, 45% of whom were retired. Among those retiring in the past year, respondents' own and spouse's retirement are rated the least stressful from a list of 31 possible events. Only 30% find retirement stressful. Retirement hassles also are less frequently reported and are rated less stressful than the work hassles of men still in the labor force. The only consistent predictors of both transitional and stage retirement stress are poor health and family finances. [2.3, 10.2]

<645> Calasanti, T. M. (1988). Participation in a dual economy and adjustment to retirement. *International Journal of Aging and Human Development*, *26*, 13-27.

Uses the white-collar/blue-collar distinction of men's placement in the world of work to examine how the economy and economic system affect retirement satisfaction. Data are a national sample of men from the NORC. Regression analyses find that placement in the work world renders two qualitatively different groups of retirees. One is primarily concerned with health (white-collar), and for the other, financial adequacy is more important for retirement adjustment. Questions about the adequacy of measurement scales to reflect the retirement transition for each group of retirees. [10.2]

<646> Campione, W. A. (1988). Predicting participation in retirement preparation programs. *Journals of Gerontology: Social Sciences*, *43*, S91-S95.

With data from the National Longitudinal Survey of Mature Men, determines the probability of participation in retirement preparation programs. It is the men who are married and have families, who have no health limitation and who have attained higher occupational status will plan for retirement. In effect, it is already those individuals who are planning for retirement who participate, and program sponsors are failing to attract a broader cross-section of employees. Concludes that the goal for the sponsors of retirement preparation programs fails to increase the voluntary participation by men (and women) who would benefit the most. [10.2]

<647> Chirikos, T. N., & Nestel, G. (1988). Work capacity of older men and age-eligibility for Medicare benefits. *Medical Care, 26,* 867-881.

Analyzes the duration of work capability of men who were middle age in 1966. Data are from the National Longitudinal Surveys of Labor Market Experience of Older Men, which includes approximately 3,500 white and 1,400 black men. Projections indicate 40 percent of the cohort of white men at age 60 are functionally capable of work at age 67, and 54 percent of those who survive until age 67 will be capable of work. Simulations for black men reveal 41 percent will be capable of work among the men who survive to age 67. Recent successive cohorts experience lower average impairment levels. Economic welfare, which will probably improve over time, should increase the capacity of men to remain working. [10.2, 12.1]

<648> Chirikos, T. N., & Nestel, G. (1991). Occupational differences in the ability of men to delay retirement. *Journal of Human Resources, 26,* 1-26.

Recognizes that the interplay between occupational assignment and the functional capacity of older men to remain at work is important to judging policies designed to change the age of retirement. Develops risk models of retirement, disability and death, and finds physical job requirements and health conditions affect the likelihood of retiring. Projections of older workers in physically strenuous and sedentary job categories that are likely to encounter difficulty in staying in the labor force do not differ greatly. Concludes with a discussion of policy considerations. [2.1, 10.2, 12.1]

<649> Danigelis, N. L., & McIntosh, B. R. (1993). Resources and the productive activity of elders: Race and gender as contexts. *Journals of Gerontology: Social Sciences, 48,* S192-S203.

Using the 1986 Amercians' Changing Lives Survey, finds in the sample of 390 white men, 161 black men, 764 white women, and 341 black women age 60 and older that individual resources (health, socioeconomic status, personal support) are dependent on both gender and race. Advantages that come with being male and white do not lead to higher productivity levels. Blacks are as at least as productive as whites, and men are significantly less productive than women. [1.4, 10.2]

<650> DeViney, S., & O'Rand, A. M. (1988). Gender-cohort succession and retirement among older men and women, 1951 to 1984. *Sociological Quarterly, 29,* 525-540.

Determines the relative influences of retirement policies and economic change on the labor force behavior of four gender-age cohorts: men age 55-64 and age 65 and older, and women aged 55-64 and aged 65 and older between 1951 and 1984. They find the structural changes in the economy have the largest impact on women and aged men. The decline in labor-force participation of men aged 65 or older is largely a response to changing demands for skills. Policies such as private employer pensions that emerge as a response to the retirement experiences of one age group become a determinant in the retirement of another, younger age group.   Due to the gender patterns in occupational distribution, changes in the pattern occupational distribution lead older males to withdraw from the labor force. Concludes that retirement is a process that transcends pension-related decisions to withdraw from work. [10.2, 12.1]

<651> Dorfman, L. T.   (1989).   Retirement preparation and retirement satisfaction in the rural elderly. *Journal of Applied Gerontology, 8,* 432-450.

Examines the relationship between preparation for retirement and retirement satisfaction. Respondents are 252 men and 199 women who participated in an 8-year epidemiological investigation of persons age 65 and over in two rural Iowa counties. Anticipatory socialization mechanisms (planning, reading about retirement, exposure to media programs about retirement) are significant in shaping retirement satisfaction. After health, planning for retirement is the second strongest predictor of retirement satisfaction for men. Gradual retirement is a correlate of satisfaction. [10.2]

<652> Dorfman, L. T.   (1992).   Academics and the transition to retirement. *Educational Gerontology, 18,* 343-363.

Interviews 104 professors to provide descriptive information on the transition from academics to retirement and to compare factors related to satisfaction before and after retirement. Finds health, rated importance of teaching, research and consulting roles, and rated importance of leisure activities are positively related to satisfaction in retirement. [10.2]

<653> Ekerdt, D. J.   (1986).   The busy ethic: Moral continuity between work and retirement. *The Gerontologist, 26,* 239-244.

Competing social constructions suggest retirement will be gratifying for the married couple or it will add strain to the marriage. Compares the marital complaints of 92 older couples where the husband was retired to 125 couples with the husband still working. Data are from the Normative Aging Study, a study of aging in community dwelling men. Similar levels of complaint are found for couples with retired men and non-retired men. These findings suggest retirement is legitimated on a day-to-day basis by a "busy ethic" that defines leisure as earnest, active, and occupied. This ethic endorses conduct that is consistent with the ideals of the work ethic. The busy ethic justifies the experience of retirement, defends retired people against judgments of senescence, and gives definition to the retirement role. It helps individuals adapt to retirement, and it in turn adapts retirement to prevailing societal values. [10.2]

<654> Ekerdt, D. J., & DeViney, S.   (1993).   Evidence for a preretirement process among older male workers. *Journals of Gerontology: Social Sciences, 48,* S35-S43.

As part of a preretirement role-exit process, older workers could be expected to reinterpret their situations and report less favorable job attitudes as they approach retirement. Using 4-wave, nine year panel data on 1,365 men age 50-69, this study shows that men evaluate their jobs as more burdensome when drawing closer to a fixed age for retirement, regardless of age and other factors. This is evidence of a preretirement dynamic, and it suggests that time-left at work organizes the experience of older workers. [10.2]

<655> Ekerdt, D. J., Vinick, B. H., & Bosse, R.   (1989).   Orderly endings: Do men know when they will retire? *Journal of Gerontology, 44,* 28-35.

Studies the timing of men's retirement relative to their own expectations from a life-course perspective. On-time and off-time retirements are assessed in a panel of older workers participating in the VA Normative Aging Study. Finds retirement is an orderly event for two-thirds of a sample who can predict and retire as planned. However, one-third of workers do not accurately foresee their date of retirement. From a practical perspective, retirement is not orderly enough when one of every three workers experiences an unscheduled exit. [10.2]

<656> Elder, G. H., & Pavalko, E. K. (1993). Work careers in men's later years: Transitions, trajectories, and historical changes. *Journals of Gerontology: Social Sciences, 48*, S180-S191.

Reviews studies depicting dramatic changes in the experience of American men at re-tirement. To investigate these changes, analyzes life history data on two birth cohorts of men in the Stanford-Terman study. Almost half of the sample (46 percent) retire gradually and nearly another third (30 percent) exit in an abrupt transition. A smaller portion (16 percent) fit a sporadic pattern of significantly reducing work or leaving the workforce and returning. Most men who exit abruptly have just one other major work-related transition in their lifetime--a promotion, a lateral move. The other retiring men previously experienced several major transitions. Cohort comparisons reveal the im-portance of broader historical forces and social changes (the depression, World War II, postwar prosperity) did not directly affect the timing or shape of retirement. [10.2]

<657> Evans, L., Ekerdt, D. J., & Bosse, R. (1985). Proximity to retirement and anticipatory involvement: Findings from the Normative Aging Study. *Journal of Gerontology, 40*, 368-374.

Examines retirement as a process, specifically whether retirement-oriented activities increase with proximity to job exit. Data are from a long-term panel study of 816 employed men. Finds preretirement involvement increased with retirement proximity and the association holds even among men who dread retirement or are satisfied with their jobs. The findings suggest that a process of anticipating retirement is underway well in advance of withdrawal from work and that a gathering involvement in retirement is normative as the event approaches. [10.2]

<658> Fletcher, W. L., & Hansson, R. O. (1991). Assessing the social components of retirement anxiety. *Psychology and Aging, 6*, 76-85.

Declares the anxiety associated with anticipated retirement ought to be viewed as a multidimensional construct. Develops the Social Components of Retirement Anxiety Scale (SCRAS) to assess the complexity of retirement anxiety in four studies involving 308 men and 384 women age 25-76. The 23-item SCRAS measures social integration and identity, social adjustment/hardiness, anticipated social exclusion, and lost friend-ships. The scale predicts fear of retirement and negative attitudes toward retirement, and finds these attitude exhibit only minimal correlations with more general measures of anxiety and depression. Elevated scores are observed particularly in persons for whom major social transitions are quite difficult--for example, those who are shy, lonely, have fewer instrumental or communal traits, or expect to have little personal control over their lives after retirement. Retirement anxiety norms do not differ for men and women of similar ages. [10.2]

<659> George, L. K., Fillenbaum, G. G., & Palmore, E. B. (1984). Sex differences in the antecedents and consequences of retirement. *Journal of Gerontology, 39,* 364-371.

Compares the antecedents and consequences of retirement among men and women. Data are from the Retirement History Study (N for analysis = 1,845) and the Duke Second Longitudinal Study (N = 235). Results suggest that known predictors of men's retirement do not predict retirement for women, and computation of the effects of retirement anticipate more of men's outcomes than women's. The only predictor of women's retirement in both samples is greater age. For men, the significant predictors of retirement include age, preretirement socioeconomic status (lower education, lower occupational status), pension coverage, various aspects of work history, health limitations, and, to a lessor extent, work-related attitudes. Retirement has positive and negative effects. It is related to perceptions of decreased health and more psychosomatic symptoms, greater self care, more time spent with friends, and increased perceptions of self-worth. Conclusions address how retirement research needs to take into consideration the fully meaning of gender. [1.1, 2.3, 10.2]

<660> Gibson, R. C. (1987). Reconceptualizing retirement for black Americans. *The Gerontologist, 27,* 660-665.

Black Americans experience work disadvantages across the life course. Four factors in combination are found in a national sample of older black Americans to contribute significantly to their unretired-retired status -- a realization that one must work from time to time well into old age, the receipt of one's income from other than private retirement pension sources, the attractiveness of and greater psychological and economic benefits of an identity as disabled rather than retired, and, most importantly, the fact that there is no clear cessation of work when the work trajectory is often disrupted. Contrary to much retirement research on whites, gender is not an important factor in the subjective retirement of blacks, since for most black men and women are lifetime workers with discontinuous work patterns. [10.2]

<661> Gibson, R. C. (1991). The subjective retirement of black Americans. *Journals of Gerontology: Social Sciences, 46,* S204-S209.

Examines why a large group of older black men and women, despite nonworking status, report themselves as not retired, and identifies causal patterns that explain subjective retirement of older blacks using data from the National Survey of Black Americans. Finds a distinct process for which older black Americans develop a retirement identity: Reluctance to define oneself as retired (subjective retirement) is sustained by perceptions of a discontinuous work life, and by the interplay among subjective disability, economic need, and psychological need for work. [10.2]

<662> Goudy, W. J., Powers, E. A., Keith, P M., & Reger, R. A. (1980). Changes in attitudes toward retirement: Evidence from a panel study of older males. *Journal of Gerontology, 35,* 942-948.

Hypothesizes and finds that as people pass through the years associated with retirement, changes in retirement attitudes tend to be small and substantively unimpressive. Data are from a panel study of 1,152 older males. Results also show that as men age, the most general attitude toward retirement as a societal consequence becomes more positive, the intermediate attitude changes hardly at all, and the most personal attitude becomes more negative. [10.2]

<663> Gustman, A. L., & Steinmeier, T. L. (1984). Partial retirement and the analysis of retirement behavior. *Industrial and Labor Relations Review, 37,* 403-415.

Finds self-reported partial retirement is relatively common in a sample of white males age 58 to 69, particularly when partial retirement is into a job different from the full-time job held earlier. Results affirm that this pattern holds even for those not facing mandatory retirement and not influenced by pension policies. [10.2]

<664> Hardy, M. A. (1991). Employment after retirement: Who gets back in? *Research on Aging, 13,* 267-288.

For some, retirement represents a transition from work to nonwork and means exit from the labor force. For others, retirement marks the beginning of a "second career" -- working full- or part-time in another job. The research examines reentry behavior using survey data from a representative sample of Florida residents. Results are supportive of a status maintenance perspective. Many of the determinants of preretirement status (race/ethnicity, gender, education) are reproduced as the predictors of unsuccessful reentry into the labor force. Not only are older men three times more likely to have postretirement employment than women, this imbalance was not reduced by introducing controls for socioeconomic status. Men, particularly white men, are characterized by higher social status during their working lives and the continue to be advantaged. [10.2]

<665> Hatch, L. R. (1992). Gender differences in orientation toward retirement from paid labor. *Gender and Society, 6,* 66-85.

Using data from the longitudinal Retirement History Study, examines orientation toward retirement in 437 previously married older women, 184 previously married older men, 120 never-married older women, and 61 never-married older men.   None of these elders are not currently married. Previously married men are more likely than previously married women to agree that older workers should retire and are more likely to define themselves as retirees.   Their economic situation is generally more advantaged. Never-married men and women do not differ on measures of retirement orientation, but they differ on a more general measure of well-being, with men holding a less positive attitude toward life in retirement. [10.1, 10.2]

<666> Haug, M. R., Belgrave, L. L., & Jones, S. (1992). Partners' health and retirement adaptation of women and their husbands. *Journal of Women and Aging, 4,* 5-29.

Examines adaptation to retirement and health among women and their husbands, where both partners are retired. Interviews 65 couples before retirement and 2 years later, after retirement. Own health and family income are indicators of adaptation for each spouse, when examined separately. But the partner's and one's own characteristics affect adaptation to retirement. A husband's chronic condition has almost as much effect on his wife's adaptation to retirement as it did on his own; by comparison, a wife's chronic condition has no impact on the adaptation of either spouse. In each couple, it is the spouse's adaptation that has the largest effect on the partner. Having a spouse happy in his or her retirement may outweigh health and money factors. [2.2, 8.4, 10.2]

<667> Hayward, M. D. (1986). The influence of occupational characteristics on men's early retirement. *Social Forces, 64*, 1032-1056.

Argues that early retirement is a function of the work context, and examines the influence of occupational characteristics on the early retirement of men. Attractiveness of an occupation is defined as the difficulties workers have in meeting task demands, the ability to derive satisfaction from the work context, and the opportunities to continue to work in a given type of job. Finds there is some age-grading of occupational "attractiveness" such that occupational characteristics gain or lose their direct salience for retirement depending on the age of incumbents. When the nature of work is controlled, the influence of pension coverage declines, suggesting that past research may have overestimated the pecuniary influence of pension benefits. [10.2]

<668> Hayward, M. D., & Grady, W. R. (1986). The occupational retention and re-cruitment of older men: The influence of structural characteristics of work. *Social Forces, 64*, 644-666.

Examines the effects of structural features of work on the occupation retention and recruitment rates of older male workers. Based on transition rates reflecting occupa-tional labor force status movements, occupational characteristics do effect movement out and in of the labor force. Movement out of the labor force and into retirement is lowest in primary sector occupations characterized by high growth, substantive complexity, and low physical demands. Reentry into the labor force is highest in secon-dary sector occupations characterized by a high concentration of elderly workers, little opportunity for skill development, few returns on seniority, and a low gap in earnings between younger and older workers. [10.2]

<669> Hayward, M. D., & Hardy, M. A. (1985). Early retirement processes among older men: Occupational differences. *Research on Aging, 7*, 491-515.

Researches the ways in which the nature of work in an occupation constrains early retirement. Using the Longitudinal Survey of Mature Men, a model of early retirement is specified in which retirement is a function of health, pension coverage, union member-ship, the wage rate, compulsory retirement regulations, tenure, and certain background factors. Finds the effects of certain traditional determinants of early retirement vary substantially across occupational work contexts. The labor force opportunities of older men are defined within an occupational context, and the impact of early retirement decisions are shaped by the nature of work. [10.2]

<670> Hayward, M. D., Grady, W. R., Hardy, M. A., & Sommers, D. G. (1989). Occupational influences on retirement, disability, and death. *Demography*,

26, 393-409.

Studies the mechanisms by which occupations directly and indirectly influence the nature and timing of older men's labor force withdrawal. Addresses the extent to which occupational factors effect exiting. Based on a hazard modeling approach, finds an occupation's task activities--substantive complexity and physical demands--are crucial aspects of the work environment that older men evaluate against nonwork alternatives. Occupational attractiveness directly effect retirement decision making. [10.2]

<671> Hayward, M. D., Crimmins, E. M., & Wray, L. A. (1994). **The relationship between retirement life cycle changes and older men's labor force participation rates.** *Journal of Gerontology: Social Sciences, 49,* S219-S230.

Examines the poor utility of using older men's labor force participation rates as an indicator of the work-to-retirement transition. The rate falsely suggest retirement is a one-time event and a permanent life status. The study illustrates a "tangled web" of behaviors underlying both labor force participation and the retirement life cycle. The authors caution against over-interpreting the historical decline in older men's labor force participation rates, for they ignore individual behavior on exiting and reentry. [10.2]

<672> Henretta, J. C., Chan, C. G., & O'Rand, A. M. (1992). **Retirement reason versus retirement process: Examining the reasons for retirement typology.** *Journals of Gerontology: Social Sciences, 47,* S1-S7.

Research often uses reasons for retirement to represent distinct paths to retirement. Critiques the conceptual basis for this retirement-reason typology, and evaluates the distinctiveness of reasons for labor force exit by trying to predict them. Data are from the 1982 Social Security New Beneficiary Study, and the analysis is limited to men. Finds the reasons for retirement just minimally capture the distinctive retirement processes. A number of other factors have distinctive effects on exit, however health limitations increase the likelihood of all types of retirement. [10.2]

<673> Herzog, A. R., Kahn, R. L., Morgan, J. N., Jackson, J. S., & Antonucci, T. C. (1989). **Age differences in productive activities.** *Journals of Gerontology: Social Sciences, 44,* S129-S138.

Determines age differences in productive contributions through both paid and unpaid work. Data are from a survey of 3,617 adults age 25 and older in 1986. Older men and women participate in many unpaid productive activities at levels that are comparable to those reached by both the middle-aged and younger adults. The activities include volunteer work in organizations, informal help to others, maintenance and repair of home, and housework. Largely because of the cessation of paid work and unpaid child care, elders spend less time overall. Men, including the group age 65 and older, spend fewer hours annually in productive activities than women their same age. [7.1, 10.2]

<674> Hooker, K., & Ventis, D. G. (1984). **Work ethic, daily activities, and retirement satisfaction.** *Journal of Gerontology, 39,* 478-484.

Suggests that both the loss of the work role and the corresponding increase in amount of unstructured time brought about by retirement could be sources of problems, particularly for retirees who value the work ethic. Relationships among retirement satisfaction, work ethic, and types of daily activities are examined in 76 retired men and women. The least satisfied retirees are those with high work values who do not perceive their activities as being useful. Men are more likely to perceive retirement as work free while women expect to continue doing the majority of the housework. Consequently, men have greater satisfaction with retirement because they could realize the ideal of retirement, a time of leisure. [10.2]

<675> Kaye, L. W., & Monk, A. (1984). Sex role traditions and retirement from academe. *The Gerontologist*, *24*, 420-426.

Literature on the differential effects of retirement for men and women in specific occupational groups is not readily available. This study documents gender differences prior to and after retirement among academics in their views of retirement planning and choice of post-retirement activities. Male retirees are most likely to continue to occupy themselves with work-oriented pursuits and more frequently assume the roles of "maintainers." Women are more apt to spend time participating in social or recreational activities and occupy "transformer" roles in retirement. Concludes that both men and women enjoy their status in retirement, despite economic strains and loss of collegial relations. [10.2]

<676> Keith, P. M. (1985). Work, retirement, and well-being among unmarried men and women. *The Gerontologist*, *25*, 410-416.

Observes an increasing proportion of aged retired population is unmarried. Investigates with longitudinal data whether 1,398 unmarrieds differ in their assessments of work, retirement, and well-being. Work is more critical to older unmarried women than to older unmarried men, and both previously married and never-married women find greater value fulfillment through work than do their male counterparts. Single men are more likely than married men to emphasize fulfillment of values through leisure compared to work, but the opposite is true for women. [2.3, 10.2]

<677> Laczko, F., Dale, A., Arber, S., & Nigel G. (1988). Early retirement in a period of high unemployment. *Journal of Social Policy*, *17*, 313-333.

Determines the reasons given by older men in England for retiring early and the extent of income poverty in early retirement. Attention is paid to how early retirement is defined and to the differences between the early retired, the sick, and the unemployed. Using data for men age 60-64 from the General Household Survey for the years 1980-1982 and from the Labour Force Survey of 1983, ill-health is a less important reason for retirement than previous studies suggest. Those who retire early are divided by class: Manual workers are more likely to retire early (because of redundancy) and, because of early retirement, more likely to be living in poverty or on very low incomes compared to nonmanual workers. [10.2]

<678> Laczko, F. (1989). Between work and retirement: Becoming 'old' in the 1980s. In B. Bytheway, T. Keil, P. Allatt, & A. Bryman (Eds.), *Becoming and*

being older: Sociological approaches to later life (pp. 24-40). London: Sage Publications.

Addresses some of the likely long term income consequences of retirement for older men and their families in England. Notes the dramatic class differences in employment rates and exit from the labor market of men (age 60-64). Just 57% of the semi- and unskilled men are employed, compared to two-thirds of the men in nonmanual occupations, despite men in the latter having greater opportunities to retire early. Most older workers retire after a period of long-term unemployment or long-term sickness; once sick, older men remain sick longer because of the increasing difficulty to reenter the labor force. The likelihood for low income in old age and experiencing poverty are markedly sharper. [10.2]

<679> Long, J. (1989).   A part to play: Men experiencing leisure through retirement. In B. Bytheway, T. Keil, P. Allatt, & A. Bryman (Eds.), *Becoming and being older: Sociological approaches to later life* (pp. 55-71). London: Sage Publications.

Academic interpretations of retirement are work-centered, with the image of retirement defined chiefly by relinquishing paid employment. It is also viewed as a stamp of old age. But retirement can mean more than the absence of work (or the presence of leisure, as leisure is defined). Viewing leisure as associated with autonomy and choice, this study examines the roles of leisure and how these shift in the transition from employment to retirement. Eight roles of leisure (e.g., keeping active, mixing socially, keeping fit, relaxing) are differentially pursued, yet remaining active seems to best suit the retired to adapt to retirement. [10.2]

<680> Martin Matthews, A., & Brown, K. H. (1987).   Retirement as a critical life event: The differential experiences of women and men. *Research on Aging, 9*, 548-571.

Much debate suggests retirement represents a crisis event, especially for men. Examines the experience of retirement among women (N = 124) and men (N = 176) living in Ontario, Canada who had been retired an average of three years. A crisis assessment determines the impact of retirement relative to other life events. Retirement, when examined in a relative sense, is a distinctly less critical life event than previous research suggests. Men are more like than women to report negative effects from retirement when the number of other life events increase. Also finds gender differences in what factors most strongly affect the experience of retirement and morale in retirement. For men, occupation-related characteristics and life-style predominate, while general health and attitude toward retirement are the most significant predictors for women. [10.2]

<681> Midanik, L. T., Soghikian, K., Ransom, L. J., & Polen, M. R. (1990).   Health status, retirement plans, and retirement: The Kaiser Permanente Retirement Study. *Journal of Aging and Health, 2*, 462-474.

Examines the stability of short-term plans to retire and the role of self-reported health status in predicting plans and actual retirement among 616 men and 446 women age 60-66 who are members of a health maintenance organization. Finds retirement plans relative stable, and accurate estimates of the age group's retirement can be made by asking. Poor health status is not related to men's plans or behavior of retirement, only women's. Rather planning for retirement and actual retirement are more closely associated with the work environment, particular having a blue-collar job. [2.4, 10.2]

<682> Morris, R., & Bass S. A. (1988). A new class in America: A revisionist view of retirement. *Social Policy, 18*, 38-43.

Theorizes that with increasing longevity, but with retirement age continuing to hover near age 65, there is a "new class" being created without a function. For the society of the 1990s, these retirees (who are predominantly men) are struggling to find a purpose or use in modern society. [10.2]

<683> Morrow-Howell, N., & Leon, J. (1988). Life-span determinants of work in retirement years. *International Journal of Aging and Human Development, 27*, 125-140.

Investigates the determinants of work effort in postretirement years. Analyzing data from the National Longitudinal Survey of Older Men, path models show that personal and structural characteristics distinguish a group of retirees who do not work the three years after retirement form those that worked more than 300 hours annually. The "retired" men who continue to participate in the labor force after retirement experience more successful employment histories before retirement. People with more marginal work histories are less likely to sustain work efforts after retirement, despite lower income. [10.2]

<684> Myers, D. A. (1991). Work after cessation of career job. *Journals of Gerontology: Social Sciences, 46*, S91-S102.

Examines the different paths wage and salary workers take into retirement using data from the Retirement History Study, and finds four distinct patterns of post-employment behavior. Higher market wages increase the probability of full-time re-employment, and wealth reduces the probability of this type of employment. Employer pension benefits greatly reduce the probability of any type of labor market participation, while Social Security benefits increase in the likelihood of partial retirement and part-time work. Results imply that recently proposed and enacted policy to discourage early retirement will have little effect on the retirement decision. [10.2]

<685> O'Rand, A. M., Henretta, J. C., & Krecker, M. L. (1992). Family pathways to retirement. In M. Szinovacz, D. J. Ekerdt, & B. H. Vinick (Eds.), *Families and retirement* (pp. 81-98). Newbury Park, CA: Sage Publications.

Contributes an interactive model to the study of retirement. Recognizes that work and family involvement exert reciprocal influences, and hypothesizes such experiences also exert indirect as well as direct influences on individual psychological functioning. Using data from the women's sample of the 1982 New Beneficiary Study, finds the paths dual-income couples follow to retirement are diverse, complex, and high contingent. Retirement is a family phenomenon, affected more by patterns of constraint than choice. Health, limited earnings and pensions, and family obligations converge to differentially constrain retirement decisions in the direction of sequential husband then wife retirement. [8.4, 10.2]

<686> Palmore, E. B., Fillenbaum, G. G., & George, L. K. (1984). Consequences of retirement. *Journal of Gerontology, 39,* **109-116.**

Examines in six longitudinal data sets the consequences of retirement, and determines if crisis or continuity theory best fits. Most research on the consequences of retirement is limited to cross-sectional data and cannot address what consequences of retirement arise when relevant preretirement activities are controlled. Finds about one-half to three-fourths of the income difference between retired and working men is caused directly by retirement; little of the observed health differences are caused by retirement; and, finds few effects of retirement on social activity, life satisfaction and happiness. These results show retirement has different effects depending on timing of retirement and type of outcome. Early retirement has stronger effects than retirement at normal ages. [10.2]

<687> Parnes, H. S., & Sommers, D. G. (1994). Shunning retirement: Work experience of men in their seventies and early eighties. *Journals of Gerontology: Social Sciences, 49,* **S117-S124.**

Examines the character of the work experience of men who continue labor force participation beyond the conventional retirement age. Data are from the National Longitudinal Surveys of Older Men. A sizable minority (16 percent) of men in their 70s and early 80s remain economically active on part- or full-time basis. The proportion declines with age -- 20 percent for men age 69-74 and 12 percent for those age 75 and older. Good health and a strong work ethic (psychological commitment to work and a corresponding distaste for retirement) are among the most important predictors of continued employment. Probability of working is also related to level of education and being married to a working wife, and negatively related to age and level of income. Of the men not working, very few gave evidence of a desire to do so. [10.2]

<688> Parsons, D. O. (1991). Male retirement behavior in the United States, 1930-1950. *Journal of Economic History, 51,* **657-670.**

Explanations for the dramatic decline in labor force participation of older men remain controversial, and include and income/wealth effect, the introduction of Old Age and Survivors Insurance, and the growth in private pension programs. Estimates from aggregate data from states suggest the means-tested Old Age Assistance program established by the Social Security Act of 1935 does significantly increase retirement activity, particularly among low-income individuals. [10.2]

<689> Ransom, R. L., & Sutch, R. (1986). The labor of older Americans: Retirement of men on and off the job, 1870-1937. *Journal of Economic History, 46,* **1-30.**

Conventional wisdom holds that 19th-century Americans worked until they died. Estimates labor force participation rates for American men sixty and over for the period 1870 through 1937. These rates suggest a higher frequency of retirement than previously anticipated and quite different trends in the incidence of retirement than commonly supposed. Evidence is also presented to establish that many older industrial workers changed to less remunerative and less demanding occupations late in their working life. This pattern of "on-the-job retirement" may have made the transition from full employment to full retirement less sudden than today. It may also reflect the lack of pensions in earlier period. [10.2, 6.2]

<690> Richardson, V., & Kilty, K. M. (1991). Adjustment to retirement: Continuity vs. discontinuity. *International Journal of Aging and Human Development*, *33*, 151-169.

Investigates the gender differences in 114 men's and 108 women's adjustment to the first year of retirement. At six months, there is an initial decline in well-being and satisfaction with relationships, more so for men than women; at one-year, both well-being and satisfaction with social contracts rebounds back, suggesting a dynamic view of adjustment to retirement is necessary. Minimal gender differences are found. Adjustment depends on the maintenance of status, income, health, and relationships. [10.2]

<691> Ruhm, C. J. (1989) Why older Americans stop working. *The Gerontologist*, *29*, 294-299.

Researchers suggest that most persons respond to economic incentives in choosing when to retire, although a small percentage of retirees exit the labor force because of deteriorating health. Recent and proposed changes in the Social Security system are incentives to remain in the labor force, and are likely to have only small effects on retirement decisions. Larger impacts are more likely to follow from altering the incentives in many private pension plans. Concludes with warning that little is known about the transition process which follows the end of career jobs and precedes retirement. [10.2, 12.1]

<692> Ruhm, C. J. (1990). Bridge jobs and partial retirement. *Journal of Labor Economics*, *8*, 482-501.

The "job-stopping" process of older workers often includes some combination of postcareer bridge employment, partial retirement, and reverse retirement. Postcareer employment is frequently outside the industry and occupation of the career job. The author finds men are less likely to remain in their career industry in a postcareer bridge job than women, men are more likely to reverse partial retirement, and men less often reenter the labor force after fully retiring. These patterns are attributed to gender differences important labor force experiences, income, and pension status. [10.2]

<693> Schuller, T. (1989). Work-ending: Employment and ambiguity in later life. In B. Bytheway, T. Keil, P. Allatt, & A. Bryman (Eds.), *Becoming and being older: Sociological approaches to later life* (pp. 41-54). London: Sage Publications.

Calls to question the image of a single prolonged stretch of continuous employment as the more. This male paradigm is being replaced by one which makes the experience of most women the norm. This feminization of employment involves the fragmentation and discontinuity of employment, the absence of a predictable occupational future, a high incidence of downward occupational mobility, involvement in part-time work, and high ambiguity for those not involved in formal employment. The collapse of the labor market for older men, combined with the trend to greater longevity, changes the picture of the life cycle. The generation of men currently finishing their working lives may be the last to exhibit the masculine work career pattern--decades of full-time employment followed by a few years or months of retirement. [1.1, 1.4, 10.2]

<694> Seccombe, K., & Lee, G. R. (1986). Gender differences in retirement satisfaction and its antecedents. *Research on Aging, 8,* 426-440.

Examines the differences between men and women in levels of self-reported satisfaction with retirement, and gender differences in the selected antecedents of retirement satisfaction--health, marital status, occupational status, and income. Using data from 1530 retired residents of Washington, finds retirement is not a markedly different experience for women and men. Retirement satisfaction seems responsive to the same causes regardless of gender. Higher-status workers appear more satisfied with retirement because they have higher incomes and better health. The lower level of satisfaction reported among women appears to be due to their lower incomes in retirement and, to a lesser extent, their lower probabilities of being married. [10.2]

<695> Swan, G. E., Dame, A., & Carmelli, D. (1991). Involuntary retirement, Type A behavior, and current functioning in elderly men: 27-year follow-up of the Western Collaborative Group Study. *Psychology & Aging, 6,* 384-391.

Examines the health and mental health consequences for voluntarily v. involuntarily retirement among 1,103 community-dwelling elder men who are either Type A personality or not. Men whose retirement is involuntary tend to have poorer adjustment to retirement, more illness, poorer physical status, and more depressive symptomatology. Type A subjects, determined both at intake (1960-1961) and at follow-up (1986-1987), report more frequent involuntary retirement. Nonetheless, minimal evidence is found to argue that Type As who retire involuntarily fare worse in retirement than those who retire voluntarily. [2.3, 10.2]

<696> Szinovacz, M. (1992). Social activities and retirement adaptation: Gender and family variations. In M. Szinovacz, D. J. Ekerdt, & B. H. Vinick (Eds.), *Families and retirement* (pp. 236-253). Newbury Park, CA: Sage Publications.

Tests the assumption that gender, marital status, and household composition determine opportunities for and set limitations on postretirement social activities. Based on a sample of 451 retired men and 376 retired women, the unmarried men are particularly involved in informal activities--visiting friends. They consolidate their network, which is somewhat isolated from kin. Married men rely more exclusively on their marriage, engage in a moderate level of activity, and exhibit low involvement in visiting with friends. Further, health problems have a significant negative effect on postretirement with friends and formal social activities. [7.1, 10.2]

<697> **Szinovacz, M., & Washo, C. (1992). Gender differences in exposure to life events and adaptation to retirement.** *Journals of Gerontology: Social Sciences, 47,* **S191-S196.**

Investigates gender differences in the experience of life events surrounding the retirement transition, and the effects such life event experiences have on adjustment to retirement. Data are from a sample of retirees covered by Florida's State Retirement System (N = 452 women and 378 men). Men report fewer life events than women during the period preceding retirement, and men's retirement adaptation are not as affected as women by the experience of life events. [1.1, 10.2]

<698> **Vinick, B. H., & Ekerdt, D. J. (1992). Couples view retirement activities: Expectation versus experience. In M. Szinovacz, D. J. Ekerdt, & B. H. Vinick (Eds.),** *Families and retirement* **(pp. 129-144). Newbury Park, CA: Sage Publications.**

Theorizes that prior to a life-course transition people think about it and try to imagine what life will be like afterward. Examines the expectations husbands and wives have toward changes in personal and couple activities after retirement. Finds 80 percent of the men and women in husband-working couples anticipate changes in activities after retirement, yet just 52 percent men and 47 percent women in husband-retired couples report an increase. Just 27 percent of husbands and 31 percent of wives in wife-working couples report an increase. These findings show expectations for changes will not be realized. [7.1, 8.4, 10.2]

<699> **Warr, P. (1992). Age and occupational well-being.** *Psychology and Aging,* **7, 37-45.**

Many studies show older workers feel more positively about the jobs than younger workers. This research examines two issues using 1,686 people in a wide range of jobs. First, there is the U-shaped relationship between age and occupational well-being (job anxiety-contentment, job depression-enthusiasm), such that middle-aged workers report lower well-being. Second, age remains significantly predictive of well-being after gender and twelve other factors are control. [2.3, 10.2]

<700> **Zsembik, B. A., & Singer, A. (1990). The problem of defining retirement among minorities: The Mexican Americans.** *The Gerontologist, 30,* **749-757.**

Of interest is the retirement process among Hispanic groups, which has received minimal attention. Uses the 1979 Chicano Survey and several operational definitions of retirement. The authors examine effects of age, gender, health, birthplace, and lifetime work experience on the meaning of retirement. Mexican American men are more likely than women to be retired when retirement is objectively defined as the receipt of a pension. However, when it is defined as an activity status, men are five times more likely to describe their activity as not retired. Social norms may prohibit these men from not working unless they are physically unable to do so. [10.2]

11

Living Arrangements

— ♦ —

LONG-TERM CARE

<701> Braun, K. L., Rose, C. L., & Finch, M. D. (1991). Patient characteristics and outcomes in institutional and community long-term care. *The Gerontologist, 31*, 648-656.

Studies who is served by what long-term care settings. Examined are the relationships among type of care (admission to a nursing home or community setting), patient characteristics, and six-month outcomes for 352 long-term care patients. A selection bias exists for the patients who enter nursing homes v. community independent-care-facility settings. If patients were placed in the opposite setting, they would not have fared any differently, thus neither setting provided patients an advantage. Concludes patient characteristics affect outcomes. After controlling for disability and diagnostic category, men appeared to do worse in both settings. [11.1]

<702> Bullard-Poe, L., Powell, C., & Mulligan, T. (1994). The importance of intimacy to men living in a nursing home. *Archives of Sexual Behavior, 23,* 231-236.

Explores the contribution of intimacy to life satisfaction among institutionalized 45 elder men who are residents of a Veterans Affairs nursing home. Rating the importance of different forms of intimacy in vignettes depicting older men in difference situations (recent admission to nursing home, notification of diagnosis of terminal illness), men identify all forms of intimacy, except sexual-physical, as important. Social intimacy is most important, followed by nonsexual physical, intellectual, and emotional. Ratings of own intimacy experiences are significantly related to the men's quality of life. [2.3, 7.1, 11.1]

<703> Cohen-Mansfield, J., & Marx, M. S. (1992). The social network of the agitated nursing home resident. *Research on Aging, 14,* 110-123.

Theorizes that agitation is not a cluster of unrelated behaviors but a set of behaviors that tend to co-occur, and these behaviors present serious management problems in the nursing home. Compares syndromes of agitation (aggressive, physically nonaggressive, verbal) to dimensions of the social network (intimacy, size/density) in 408 nursing home residents. Shows that men are more disruptive, and the social networks of aggressive residents and verbally agitated residents lack intimacy. Network size/density does not differentiate among residents. [7.5, 11.1]

<704> Kaye, L. W., & Monk, A. (1991). Social relations in enriched housing for the aged: A case study. *Journal of Housing for the Elderly, 9* (1-2), 111-126.

Examines the influence of progressive aging on the social lives of 210 elderly tenants of two housing facilities. Finds a lack of symmetry in assistance exchanges between elders and their relatives, who are more likely to assist the elders than the reverse; however, symmetry is apparent with externally residing friends as well as fellow tenants. Men and residents over 75 received less assistance. Also findings the number of available social supports (e.g., children, grandchildren, friends, and fellow tenants) is positively correlated with satisfaction with life. [8.1, 11.1]

<705> Spector, W. D., & Jackson, M. E. (1994). Correlates of disruptive behaviors in nursing homes: A reanalysis. *Journal of Aging and Health, 6,* 173-184.

Examines factors associated with the occurrence of disruptive behaviors (abusive behavior, wandering, noisiness) among 3,351 nursing home residents from 103 certified nursing homes in Rhode Island. The authors find the likelihood of exhibiting disruptive behavior increases with severity of both cognitive and functional impairment, and decreases with immobility. Men are more likely to be abusive, whereas no gender effects are noted for wandering or being noisy. In contrast to earlier reports, age and communication problems are not related to disruptiveness. [2.1, 11.1]

<706> Tesch, S. A., Nehrke, M. F., & Whitbourne, S. K. (1989). Social relation-ships, psychological adaptation, and intrainstitutional relocation of elderly men. *The Gerontologist, 29,* 517-523.

Theorizes the movement of an intact population of institutionalized elderly might be less disruptive of the social environment than relocation of individuals. Investigates the social interaction and the self-report and behavioral measures of psychological adapta-tion of 40 men age 53 to 91 before and after an involuntary intrainstitutional relocation. Finds the relocated men score lower on a morale scale assessing attitudes toward aging, have fewer peer friends within the institution and lower friendship scores, yet evidence better communication (or interacted more with staff following relocation) than do unrelocated men. The negative effect of the move is greater on men who have larger social networks than the more socially isolated men. Presence of a peer confi-dant after the move is not directly related to morale, perhaps because an elderly friend in failing health is as much a worrisome responsibility as a source of personal support. [2.3, 7.5, 11.1]

<707> Valliant, P. M., & Furac, C. J. (1993). Type of housing and emotional health of senior citizens. *Psychological Reports, 73,* 1347-1353.

Correlations among three housing conditions -- detached unit, multi-unit, institution -- and scores for depression, self-esteem, and anxiety are examined for 85 men and women age 50 and older. Analyses indicate that men residing within an institution are significantly more depressed than those residing within detached homes, and they are significantly more depressed than women in both situations. There are no significant differences associated with type of residence and measures of anxiety or self-esteem. [2.3, 11.1]

COMMUNITY RESIDENCE

<708> Alexander, F., & Duff, R. (1988). Social interaction and alcohol use in retirement communities. *The Gerontologist, 28*, 632-636.

Recognizes that retirement communities are often portrayed as involving leisure-oriented, socially active lifestyles. Surveys residents of three retirement communities and finds regular drinking is more common in these communities than in the general population of elders. Drinking is associated with greater social activity, not isolation or the stresses of aging. Gender is predictive--men drink more than women, in keeping with the cultural norm. Outside activities or the visiting of children do not alter the relation between socializing and alcohol use. The social life of the communities socialize elders to associate drinking as a social ritual. [4.2, 7.1, 11.2]

<709> Burr, J. A. (1990). Race/sex comparisons of elderly living arrangements: Factors influencing the institutionalization of the unmarried. *Research on Aging, 12*, 507-530.

Summarizes trends in the institutionalization rates of unmarried black and white elders, and analyzes the individual attributes associated with the probability of institutionalization. Using the 1960-1980 Census, there convergence appears in age-standardized rates across both race and gender. Married white men compared to unmarried women and blacks are increasing their use of institutions at faster paces to make all population groups more alike in institutionalization rates. This means considerable consistency in which economic and health factors predict the likelihood of being in a long-term care setting. [11.2]

<710> Chappell, N. L. (1991). Living arrangements and sources of caregiving. *Journals of Gerontology: Social Sciences, 46*, S1-S8.

Investigates whether living with someone is more important for caregiving than the exact relationship. Confirms prior findings that married people tend to receive assistance from their spouse; however, it is the structural characteristic of living with someone, rather than marital status, which is important for receiving instrumental care. Among older men, the married men identify their spouse as a preferred caregiver more often than married women, perhaps because older men's spouses are younger and healthier. Men and women are as likely to name their spouse when they are already serving as the primary caregiver. [7.5, 9.2, 11.2]

<711> Coward, R. T., & Cutler, S. J. (1991). The composition of multigenerational households that include elders. *Research on Aging, 13,* 55-73.

Reports that prior findings show one in five elders resided in multigenerational households, and examines in detail the composition of two- and three-or-more generation households. Finds more elders reside with consanguine kin than with in-laws. As age increases, a higher percentage of elders live with their children, grandchildren, or kin who are not spouses or siblings. In two-generation families, there is a steady decline in the percent older men and women who live with a son and an increase who live with a daughter. Unmarried children, especially sons, are more likely to share the household. [8.2, 11.2]

<712> Coward, R. T., Cutler, S. J., & Schmidt, F. E. (1989). Differences in the household composition of elders by age, gender, and area of residence. *The Gerontologist, 29,* 814-821.

Examines the relationships of elders to other household members for age, gender, and area-of-residence differences in household types and generational composition. Determines that the majority elders live in some form of family household; most prevalent are two-person, married-couple-only households at age 65-79. Men are twice as likely to be living in the married-couple-only household, and women are more apt than men to be living alone, especially with advancing age. One in five elders lives in a household comprised of more than one generation, and three-quarters of these are in two generation only arrangements. Although some gender differences in multigenerational living can be found, advanced age is the greatest determinant. [11.2]

<713> Crimmins, E. M., & Ingegneri, D. G. (1990). Interaction and living arrangements of older parents and their children. *Research on Aging, 12,* 3-35.

Examines the effect of social, economic, and demographic changes on likelihood of an elders living with a child. Analyses are based n the 1984 National Health Interview Survey Study on Aging and the 1962 and 1975 Survey of the Aged studies. Finds that without controlling for other factors (such as marital status), one might conclude that more women live with their children. But multivariate analyses show that men are more likely than women to live with a son or daughter. The likelihood increases if the child is unmarried and without the competing demands of a family. [8.2, 11.2]

<714> Davis, M. A., Neuhaus, J. M., Moritz, D, J., & Segal, M. R. (1992). Living arrangements and survival among middle-aged and older adults in the NHANES-I epidemiologic follow-up study. *American Journal of Public Health, 82,* 401-406.

Examines how living alone affects the health and survival of older adults with data on 7,651 older adults. Notes that by 1990, approximately 30 percent of elders lived alone, yet just one-fifth of these solitary elders were men. Nonetheless, there is a stronger association between living alone and being disadvantaged in terms of survival for men than for women, and for middle-aged men than for older men. Those living alone and those living with someone other than a spouse are equally at a higher risk of mortality. The findings suggest that living arrangements have no additional influence on mortality beyond marital status. [2.1, 11.2]

<715> De Vos, S. (1990). **Extended family living among older people in six Latin American countries.** *Journals of Gerontology: Social Sciences, 45,* S87-S94.

Compares the sociodemographic underpinnings for older adults living in an extended family in Columbia, Costa Rica, Dominican Republic, Mexico, Panama, and Peru. In contrast to Western countries, the majority of elders live in extended family households, and unmarried elders are especially included. Unmarried men are less likely than women to live in the extended family, perhaps because of the traditionally of being more economically independent. Concludes that there is little or no relationship among extended family living and age or urban/rural residence in the countries studied. [11.2]

<716> Dolinsky, A. L., & Rosenwaike, I. (1988). **The role of demographic factors in the institutionalization of the elderly.** *Research on Aging, 10,* 235-257.

Determines the relationship between demographic factors and institutionalization of the very old. Using the 1980 census, attention is given to the role of close kin, especially spouses and children, in reducing the risk of institutionalization. Associated with institutionalization are the absence of a spouse and child, advanced age, and presence of disability. Less expected is the significance of marital status for men relative to women. Concludes elderly men are more dependent than their female counterparts, and these men are typically older and have greater disability. [9.1, 11.2]

<717> Elias, C. J., & Inui, T. S. (1993). **When a house is not a home: Exploring the meaning of shelter among chronically homeless older men.** *The Gerontologist, 33,* 396-402.

Explores the social world of 35 chronically homeless older men in Seattle, especially their experience with sheltered living and its effect on health-seeking behavior. For many, the shelter provides a sanctuary in a world of loneliness and addiction--a place of safety, support, community--but only temporarily. Public shelters' merry-go-round timetable require the older man to move to the streets each morning, to return at evening. This timetable contributes to how men forfeit their sense of responsibility to a routine. In this case, their capacity for self-care erodes, utilization of services declines, alcohol use and "giving up" increases, and they become dependent on outreach and rescue efforts. [2.3, 4.2, 10.1, 11.2]

<718> Ford, A. B., Roy, A. W., Haug, M. R., Folmar, S. J., & Jones, P. K. (1991). **Impaired and disabled elderly in the community.** *American Journal of Public Health, 81,* 1207-1209.

Reports information about the distribution between community and long-term institutional care over a nine-year period for a representative sample of 1,598 urban elderly. Of the survivors in 1984, age 74 and older, finds just 11 percent had been admitted to long-term care for 30 days or more. Of the persons who died, however, finds 28 percent listed a nursing home as the usual residence at death. Socioeconomic advantage--younger age, male gender, better income, and living with others, especially children--favors continuing care in the home. [11.1, 11.2]

<719> Freedman, V. A., Berkman, L. F., Rapp, S. R., & Ostfeld, A. M. (1994). Family networks: Predictors of nursing home entry. *American Journal of Public Health, 84*, 843-845.

Despite the theoretical and practical importance of kin in caring for older relatives, few studies examine the relationship between the family network and the risk of nursing home placement. Data from a cohort of noninstitutionalized elderly persons in New Haven in 1982 reveal that older persons who have regular contact with kin have a lower risk of institutionalization. For men, the spouse is most important in reducing the risk. [9.2, 11.2]

<720> Hanley, R. J., Alecxih, L. M. B., Wiener, J. M., & Kennell, D. L. (1990). Predicting elderly nursing home admissions: Results from the 1982-84 National Long-Term Care Survey. *Research on Aging, 12*, 199-228.

Rapidly growing demands for long-term care strain public and private resources. This work is designed to improve the ability to predict institutionalization of disabled elders, and it finds among predictors of nursing home admissions that age and health factors are crucial. Unanticipated, income and asset wealth are nonsignificant predictors of admission. Neither is gender a predictor, when controlling for other variables, even though men constitute the minority of residents. [11.2]

<721> Lieberman, M. A., & Kramer, J. H. (1991). Factors affecting decisions to institutionalize demented elderly. *The Gerontologist, 31*, 371-374.

Follows 321 community-dwelling patients with dementia, nearly one-quarter (22%) of whom are institutionalized after one year. Analysis indicate that, with one exception, none of the patient characteristics, such as gender or level of impairment, predict institutionalization. The exception is patients without a spouse are consistently found to be a greater risk for institutionalization (which suggests older women who outlive caregiving husbands are at greater risk). Institutionalization is associated more with the caregiving situation--the greater the number of family members and friends involved and/or the greater the caregiver distress, the more likely institutionalization occurs. [9.2, 11.2]

<722> Mittelman, M. S., Ferris, S. H., Steinberg, G., Shulman, E., Mackell, J. A., Ambinder, A., & Cohen, J. (1993). An intervention that delays institutionalization of Alzheimer's disease patients: Treatment of spouse-caregivers. *The Gerontologist, 33*, 730-740.

Spouse caregivers are randomly assigned to either a treatment group (individual and family counseling, support group participation, and ad hoc consultation) or a control group involving only routine support. In the first year the treatment group has less than half as many nursing home placements. No greater the risk of placement is found when the caregivers are husbands, rather placement is affected by patient's lower income conferring greater odds and the patient's need for assistance with activities of daily living. Concludes with the observation that counseling in behalf of caregivers reduces the risks of placement. [8.4, 9.1, 11.2]

<723> Montgomery, R. J. V., & Kosloski, K. (1994). A longitudinal analysis of nursing home placement for dependent elders cared for by spouses vs adult children. *Journals of Gerontology: Social Sciences, 49*, S62-S74.

Addresses predictors of nursing home placement in the context of who provides informal care within the family. Panel data from 531 caregivers and their frail elders are analyzed to identify how changes in the caregiving situation are related to nursing home placement. Men more often reach the decision to institutionalize. For spouse caregivers, particularly husbands, it is the subjective burden which helps trigger placement, whereas for adult children it is the objective burden. The trajectory for institutionalization is much different for adult children than spouses, rising sharply near the two-year mark of caregiving. These differences between spouse and adult children may reflect differences in when and how caregiving formally begins, since spouses assume many caregiving tasks as a normal part of the marital role and the process of self-definition as a caregiver may take a much longer period of time. [9.2, 11.2]

<724> Reitzes, D. C., Mutran, E., & Pope, H. (1991). Location and well-being among retired men. *Journals of Gerontology: Social Sciences, 46*, S195-S203.

With the "graying of the suburbs" there is a need to understand if residential location has an impact on the well-being of elders. Data are from a national sample of retired men age 60-74. Findings suggest location produces differences in well-being, with retired men living in suburbs having the highest mean well-being scores; poor health reduces the well-being of retired men in the suburbs to a greater extent than in the central cities; and suburban location also indirectly influences well-being by way of its effect on informal activities. [2.3, 11.2]

<725> Stinner, W. F., Byun, Y., & Paita, L. (1990). Disability and living arrangements among elderly American men. *Research on Aging, 12*, 339-363.

The living arrangements of disabled elders affect public policy issues. This study tests four models of ways in which disability might affect coresidence with adult relatives. Uses the 1976 and 1981 panels of the National Longitudinal Survey of Mature Men, and finds men with multiple disabling conditions, not a single disability, are more likely to live with adult relatives than nondisabled men. The absence of a spouse may reinforce this pattern. [2.1, 11.2, 12.1]

<726> Tell, E. J., Cohen, M. A., Larson, M. J., & Batten, H. L. (1987). Assessing the elderly's preferences for lifecare retirement options. *The Gerontologist, 27*, 503-509.

Elders needing long-term care continue to become more noticeable. Among applicants to two retirement communities, the older men express more interest in care at home than either women or younger male applicants. The older men are more interested in community living and more resistant to a lifestyle change. Although they make application, their commitment to moving appears weaker than their younger counterparts. By comparison, applicants seeking membership in the retirement communities for social rather than health or financial reasons are uninterested in care at home. Surprisingly, this group included married men. Several masculinity hypotheses are presented as possible explanations. [11.2]

<727> Worobey, J. L., & Angel, R. J. (1990). Functional capacity and living arrangements of unmarried elderly persons. *Journals of Gerontology: Social Sciences, 45*, S95-S101.

Uses the 1986 Longitudinal Study of Aging and examines the impact of gender, race and ethnicity, functional capacity, and various socioeconomic characteristics on changes in living arrangements among unmarried elders. Even when they experience significant declines in health, most single elderly persons who live alone at the initial interview continue to live alone two years later. It is the decline in functional capacity that greatly increases the likelihood an elderly person will move in with others or become institutionalized. Multivariate analysis shows men who suffer declines in functional capacity are somewhat more likely than women to be unable to live alone. [2.1, 11.2]

12

Resources and Needs

—◆—

POLICY CONSIDERATIONS

<728> Arber, S., & Ginn, J. (1991). *Gender and later life: A sociological analysis of resources and constraints.* Newbury Park, CA: Sage Publications.

Addresses the importance of gender among elders. An overview is presented of the demographic changes in Great Britain and the United States that have resulted in an aging population and the gender imbalance as age advances. Age discrimination is examined in relation to older people generally, but toward older women specifically. Three key resources are shown to form an interlocking triangle: financial and material circumstances, health, and access to domestic and personal care. Each of these resources is examined regarding the extent of elderly women's disadvantage compared with elderly men and its implications. [1.1, 10.1, 12.1]

<729> Chirikos, T. N., & Nestel, G. (1989). **Occupation, impaired health, and the functional capacity of men to continue working.** *Research on Aging,* **11,** 174-205.

Analyzes whether the functional capacity of older men to remain at work differs by occupational assignment, and discusses its importance in judging policies designed to advance the age of retirement. Data are on a nationally representative sample. Finds workers in either physically demanding or sedentary jobs who retire nondisabled are very similar. Health conditions play an important role in determining the ability of the men to delay retirement, however the nature of the work also plays an important role. Physical job requirements and health condition jointly affect the likelihood of retiring in a disabled state. Policy consideration of workers in physically demanding occupations may be questioned. [1.4, 12.1]

<730> Clark, D. O., & Maddox, G. L. (1992). **Social context and personal expenditures for health care: Federal policy and the experience of older adults in the 1970s.** *Journal of Aging and Social Policy,* **4,** 179-198.

Determines the effects of federal income and health care reimbursement policies in the late 1960s and early 1970s on health care behavior and expenditures in the decade

1970-1980. Data from the Longitudinal Retirement History Study confirm the anticipated effects of increasing age and expanded insurance coverage (Medicare/Medicaid): There is an increase in health care expenditures and a decrease in the relative burden of out-of-pocket health care costs. The data support the view that access to care for the elderly expanded during the 1970s. Results also show that low-income persons pay a higher proportion of their income for health care than do other subgroups. Universal coverage programs that incorporate high out-of-pocket costs are likely to negatively affect the utilization rates of low-income groups, unless reimbursement schedules are set according to the ability to pay. [12.2, 12.1]

<731> Dressel, P. (1988). Gender, race, and class: Beyond the feminization of poverty in later life. *The Gerontologist, 28,* 177-180.

Does not debate that argument that patriarchy creates significant burdens for older women. Nor debated is whether one form of inequality is more oppressive than another. Rather, contends that as appealing as the feminization of poverty argument may be to age-based and women's advocacy, it has the potential for oversimplifying the issue of old age poverty, and the potential for being politically divisive. The singular focus on one gender ignores the diversity within gender and the similarities across gender. For example, the median income from Social Security for non-married black men is less than for non-married white women, and non-married black men are more likely (64 percent) to fall below a poverty mark than non-married white women (49 percent). In the feminization argument the racial-ethnic men's systematic marginality is ignored. [10.1, 12.1]

<732> Gonyea, J. G. (1994). Making gender visible in public policy. In E. Thompson (Ed.), *Older men's lives* (pp. 237-255). Thousand Oaks, CA: Sage Publications.

Examines one macro-micro interaction of gender and aging -- how public policies differential influence the well-being of elders. Begins with fundamental sociological premise that gender is a relational construct, and definitions of masculinity and manhood reveal institutionalized advantages benefiting older men, whether the focus is economic status and risk of poverty, marital status and the risk of loneliness or institutionalization, or work-life experience and sources of income in later life. Reviews how Social Security and the Supplemental Security Income Program both were designed for the white, single-earner family and now benefit men more than women, and white, middle-class men more than other men. Concludes that greater gender and age equity requires redesigning public policy and programs. [10.1, 12.1]

<733> Kahne, H. (1985-86). Not yet equal: Employment experience of older women and older men. *International Journal of Aging and Human Development, 22,* 1-13.

Discusses the consistency of patterns of gender inequality and how older men's employment-related experience is more frequently advantaged. Reviews six ways men's employment-related experiences differ from that of women: labor force participation rates, occupational distribution, earnings, unemployment, poverty, and retirement income. Concludes the review addressing a number of suggestions for policy which would markedly improve the status of older women to compare with the status of men. [10.2, 12.1]

<734> Quadagno, J., Meyer, M. D., & Turner, J. B. (1991). Falling into the Medicaid gap: The hidden long-term care dilemma. *The Gerontologist, 31,* 521-526.

Examines descriptively older Florida residents who fall into the Medicaid gap -- those whose incomes are too high to obtain eligibility for Medicaid yet too low to cover the costs of nursing home care as private pay patients. Those most likely to fall into the gap are individuals with continuous work histories and those who have worked long enough to qualify for a pension. They are more likely to be men. It is these men's primary caregivers, their wives and children, who face the financial and emotional caregiving burden when the men are deemed ineligible for Medicaid. [9.1, 10.1, 12.1]

<735> Snell, J. G. (1993). Gendered construction of elderly marriage, 1900-1950. *Canadian Journal on Aging, 12,* 509-523.

Canadian state policies in the 1930s and 1940s addressing the old-age pension program reveal a systemic bias in the way the programmed maintained the traditional, gendered hierarchy of power in elderly marriages. The author discusses how the Canadian state's decision to provide direct aid to the elderly on the basis of need is undermined by its assumptions about the gendered character of marriage. [6.2, 12.1]

<736> Sorensen, A. (1991). Restructuring of gender relations in an aging society. *Acta Sociologica, 34,* 45-55.

Discusses ways in which more egalitarian gender relations between men and women in both the public and private spheres can emerge in aging societies where life expectancies are high and old people constitute a high proportion of the population. Concludes that to realize greater equality, institutional constraints on change must be overcome. [6.2, 12.1]

HEALTH CARE RESOURCES AND NEEDS

<737> Bass, D. M., Looman, W. J., & Ehrlich, P. (1992). Predicting the volume of health and social services: Integrating cognitive impairment into the modified Anderson framework. *The Gerontologist, 32,* 33-43.

Examines cognitive impairment as a predictor of the volume of community services used by older adults who were either mentally impaired or intact. Predictors of service utilization are tested with 246 social service and 97 health care clients. Gender is not predictive among health care clients; requests for and receipt of health services are more prevalent among the intact clients with burdened caregivers. Social service use varies with gender, and least frequent clients are older men who do not live alone and have secondary caregivers (most likely, their children). Contends that men caring for female clients are likely to relinquish personal care to paid providers. [2.5, 12.2]

<738> Bazargan, M., & Barbre, A. R. (1992). **Knowledge of medication use among black elderly.** *Journal of Aging and Health, 4*, 536-550.

Assesses the prevalence and correlates of mis/nonidentification of the therapeutic purpose of prescription drugs in a sample of 621 black elderly. One-third of the elders either could not identify or misidentified the purpose of at least one of their prescribed drugs. Knowledge is inversely related to number of medications prescribed. Black men who are older and report a lower level of perceived availability and accessibility to physician services are more likely to mis/nonidentify therapeutic purpose. [2.5, 12.2]

<739> Burns, B. J., Wagner, H. R., Taube, J. E., Magaziner, J., Permutt, T., & Landerman, R. (1993). **Mental health service use by the elderly in nursing homes.** *American Journal of Public Health, 83*, 331-337.

Identifies predictors of mental health service use and estimates the impact of the 1987 mandate to treat mental illness in nursing home residents--Public Law 100-203. Data are from the 1985 National Nursing Home Survey. Finds two-thirds of elderly residents had a mental disorder, but just under five percent of these patients receive mental health treatment from either a mental health professional or general physician during the past month. Gender is not a predictor for being seen by either a specialist or general practitioner, although there is a pattern for older men to be seen by a mental health specialist more than women. Findings indicate significant neglect of the mental health needs of older nursing home residents. [2.5, 12.2]

<740> Chipperfield, J. G. (1993). **Perceived barriers in coping with health problems: A twelve-year longitudinal study of survival among elderly individuals.** *Journal of Aging and Health, 5*, 123-139.

Examines the relationship between perceived barriers to health and men's and women's mortality 12 years later. Data are from the Aging in Manitoba Studies (N = 2,052 men and 2,265 women age 65 and older in 1971). Three types of perceived barriers are identified: control barriers (perceived lack of control over health and inability to manage health), personal barriers (language and memory deficits), and societal barriers (transportation and financial problems). Logistic regression analyses reveal control and personal (not societal) barriers predict mortality 12 years later as much as being a male. This finding is only predictive for elders who began the study in average or poor (rather than good) health. Concludes that the elderly individuals--particularly men--with health problems who perceive barriers to maintaining their health are more likely to die than those who do not. [2.1, 2.3, 12.2]

<741> Collison, B. B. (1987). **Counseling aging men.** In M. Scher, M. Stevens, G. Good, & G. A. Eichenfield (Eds.), *Handbook of counseling & psychotherapy with men* (pp. 165-177). Newbury Park, CA: Sage Publications.

Reviews a therapeutic technique for working with older men. The objective is to assist them in assessing their lives, to determine what their lives mean and what aging means for them, and to allow them to implement whatever they need to do as a result of the meaning that they define. [12.2]

<742> De-Ortiz, C. M. (1993). The politics of home care for the elderly poor: New York City's Medicaid-funded home program. *Medical Anthropology Quarterly, 7*, 4-29.

Examines a Medicaid-funded home health care program for the elderly in New York City. Shows that the resources available to the elderly and their health condition can only be understood in terms of the impact of class position throughout their lives. Analysis of the differences in funding by gender is also presented, with men over-benefiting. [12.2]

<743> Fredericks, C. M., te Wierik, M. J., van Rossum, H. J., Visser, A., Volovics, A., & Sturmans F. (1992). Why do elderly people seek professional home care? Methodologies compared. *Journal of Community Health, 17*, 131-141.

Investigates which characteristics, besides physical limitations, contribute to the utilization of professional home care among elders who are living at home. Based on interviews with 450 men and women age 55 and older, bivariate analysis reveals that users of professional care are older, less often men, more often not married, more often living alone, and with less extensive social networks. Simply put, amount of informal care available and household composition contribute to utilization, and because older men are more likely married and not alone, they use fewer services. [12.2]

<744> Goldsteen, R., Counte, M. A., Glandon, G. L., & Goldsteen, K. (1992). Desirable life events and physician utilization among older American men and women. *Journal of Aging Studies, 6*, 149-163.

Studies the relationship between desirable life events and outpatient physician utilization, based on interviews with 346 adults age 56-91. Finds the effect of desirable events on utilization is complex and indirect, largely due to the impact of desirable events on psychological well-being and on perception of health status. When the number of desirable life events exceeds two, the costs (in fatigue, time, and energy) reduce the benefits. [2.3, 12.2]

<745> Hansell, S., Sherman, G., & Mechanic, D. (1991). Body awareness and medical care utilization among older adults in an HMO. *Journals of Gerontology: Social Sciences, 46*, S151-S159.

Considerable attention has been given to medical care utilization among elders. This research investigates the association between body awareness and utilization among 1,124 older adult members of a health maintenance organization. In contrast to common sense wisdom, older men and women do not appreciably differ in body awareness, and those with greater body awareness have significant increases over time in the volume of patient-initiated illness visits to the HMO and hospital emergency room. In contrast, body awareness is not associated with changes in physician-initiated follow-up visits, referrals, or hospital days. [2.4, 2.5, 12.2]

<746> Haug, M. R., & Ory, M G. (1987). Issues in elderly patient-provider interactions. *Research on Aging, 9*, 3-44.

Surveys the state of knowledge concerning relationships between elderly patients and their health care providers. Finds characteristics of physicians, including age, gender, practice styles, and psychological attitudes, are relevant to the course and content of interactions. Equally critical are the characteristics of the elder patients. Concludes, however, research on interactions between providers and elderly patients is sparse, particularly the lack of research on the effects of patients' gender and race. [9.1, 12.2]

<747> High, D. M. (1990). Old and alone: Surrogate health care decision-making for the elderly without families. *Journal of Aging Studies, 4* (3), 277-288.

From in-depth interviews of 20 men and women age 65-91, investigates the surrogate health care decision-making for elderly persons who live alone and do not have families to rely on. Finds friends and physicians are the preferred surrogate resources for elderly people without families. Some participants report that they had no one on whom to rely. Findings reveal that elderly people without families have not engaged in much planning for long-term care and related health care decision-making. They hope to continue to make their own decisions and to care for themselves until the end of their lives. Professionals are urged to initiate discussions with family-less elderly concerning use of proxy appointments for future health care decisions.

<748> Hirsch, C. H., Davies, H. D., Boatwright, F., & Ochango, G. (1993). Effects of a nursing-home respite admission on veterans with advanced dementia. *The Gerontologist, 33*, 523-528.

The short-term admission to a nursing home of patients with dementia represents an important respite option for their caregivers, yet little is known about how it affects the patients. Twenty-six of 39 men admitted to a Veterans Affairs dementia respite program experience a small but significant decline in self-care and behavior at two days after discharge, but by 14 days most return to their pre-respite status. Patients who deteriorated substantially have, on average, greater independence in self-care and less cognitive impairment at admission than those who improved or worsened minimally. [2.3, 9.1, 11.1, 12.2]

<749> Keith, P. M. (1987). Postponement of health care by widowed, divorced, and never-married older men. *Lifestyles, 8* (3-4), 70-81.

Investigates relationships between marital status and postponement of health care, reasons for postponement, and changes in health care behavior from 1969 to 1979 among 375 unmarried older men. Almost 30 percent have not sought care when their health warranted it. Postponement of care is not associated with marital status (formerly or never-married), but the different reasons for foregoing care are. Discriminant analyses indicate the general importance of financial distress of postponing care. [12.2]

<750> Koenig, H. G., Bearon, L. B., & Dayringer, R. (1989). Physician perspectives on the role of religion in the physician-older patient relationship. *Journal of Family Practice, 28*, 441-448.

Studies primary care physicians' perspectives on the role of religion in the doctor-patient relationship. Most family physicians and general practitioners (N = 160) believe religion has a positive effect on the mental health of older patients, and many primary care physicians also believe religion has a favorable effect on physical health. Physicians are skeptical about religious issues being reserved completely for the clergy. Nearly 66% fell that prayer with patients is appropriate, and over 33% report having prayed with older patients during extreme physical or emotional distress. Younger physicians have positive attitudes toward addressing religious issues. [5.1, 12.2]

<751> Leszcz, M., Feigenbaum, E., Sadavoy, J., & Robinson, A. (1985). A men's group: Psychotherapy of elderly men. *International Journal of Group Psychotherapy, 35*, 177-196.

Although elderly men are thought to be nonresponsive to psychotherapy, describes a group psychotherapy intervention for 7 men age 70-95 who are living in a nursing home. Discusses strategies which facilitate men's efforts to maintain their self-esteem and sense of self while living in an institution, particularly the role of life review. [1.2, 12.2]

<752> Martin, J. P. (1990). Male cancer awareness: Impact of an employee education program. *Oncology Nursing Forum, 17*, 59-64.

Reviews how prostate cancer has surpassed lung cancer as the leading cancer in men. Encouraged by advances in ultrasound technology, early detection is more reliable, and the expansion of the aging population will increase prostate cancer threefold by the year 2030. A quasi-experimental study investigates knowledge about and attitudes toward prostate and testicular cancer among men working for an electrical power company (N = 448). Concludes that implementation of a male cancer awareness educational program would be worthwhile. [2.5, 12.2]

<753> Mutran, E., & Ferraro, K. F. (1988). Medical need and use of services among older men and women. *Journals of Gerontology: Social Sciences, 43*, S162-S171.

The additive and interactive effects of gender and gender roles affect the experience of health and health behaviors, not just the outcomes of discretionary physician visits and hospitalization. Aging acts as an equalizer of physician contacts among men and women, and poor health by itself is no more likely to cause older women to see a physician than older men. But, gender affects in the process of men's and women's help seeking: Men who assess their health as poor are more likely to see a physician than are women, and men's health is more affect by variables related to their employment such as income and education. Also, given equal levels of disability and health status, older men are more likely to be hospitalized. This differential could arise from physicians' perception of men as not willing to care for themselves and physicians having less information about the men as patients given gender differences in earlier help seeking. [12.2]

<754> Phillips, M. A., & Murrell, S. A. (1994). Impact of psychological and physical health, stressful events, and social support on subsequent mental health help seeking among older adults. *Journal of Consulting and Clinical Psychology, 62*, 270-275.

Prospectively examines factors that influence mental health help seeking among 240 adults age 55 and older. Older men have a low rate of seeking services from a physician. Instead, they visit a mental health center or clinic. Discriminant analysis separating those who do from those who do not need and seek services reveals that help seekers have poorer psychological well-being, more physical health problems, greater unpleasant stressful events, and greater deficits in social support. [2.3, 2.5, 12.2]

<755> Rakowski, W., Rice, C., & McHorney, C. A. (1992). Information-seeking about health among older adults. *Behavior, Health, and Aging*, *2*, 181-198.

An unresolved question in health behavior research is whether behaviors form empirical clusters or are largely independent. Data from a 1987-1988, two-wave panel of 487 elders age 65 and older are used to investigate information-seeking about health. Results indicate the existence of a health behavior reflecting information seeking, and it is similar for both older men and older women. This behavior is not directly influenced by age, income, or education. Results also suggest a stable health behavior across time, perhaps representing a basic self-care tendency. Information-seeking is associated with vigorous activity, checking medication expiration dates, seatbelt use, asking to sit in nonsmoking sections, and controlling exposure to sunlight. [2.5, 12.2]

<756> Rivnyak, M. H, Wan, T. T., Stegall, M. H., Jacobs, M., & Li, S. (1989). Ambulatory care use among the noninstitutionalized elderly. *Research on Aging*, *11*, 292-311.

Factors influencing health service utilization by the noninstitutonalized elderly include personal and social determinants of ambulatory care use. Uses a LISREL model to identify the extent to which ambulatory care use is affected by need, both physical and mental. Results affirm that physical dysfunction has the strongest direct, positive effect. Older men are less likely to use services than women. Elders with more psychological problems are also unlikely to use ambulatory services. [2.5, 12.2]

<757> Sharp, J. W., Blum, D., & Aviv, L. (1993). Elderly men with cancer: Social work interventions in prostate cancer. *Social Work in Health Care*, *19*, 91-107.

Argues that prostate cancer requires the attention of social workers in health care for three reasons--the growing elderly population that will increase the number diagnosed, the recent introduction of new treatments, and the lack of social acceptability for this condition. Interventions for prostate cancer are specific to the stage of the disease. These individual, family, and group interventions are a model for social work services to elderly men with other forms of cancer. Social workers have the opportunity to research quality of life and decision-making issues to enhance medical practice in prostate cancer. [2.1, 12.2]

<758> Strain, L. A. (1991). Use of health services in later life: The influences of health beliefs. *Journals of Gerontology: Social Sciences*, *46*, S143-S150.

Increasing attention in health care has spotlighted the elderly as the largest group of adult users of services. Unknown is whether service use is based on need or other factors. This work examines the influence of health beliefs on use of health services by 743 adult Canadians age 60 and older. The analysis is based on Andersen-Newman's model of predisposing, enabling, and need factors affecting utilization. Need emerges as the strongest correlates of physician visits, hospitalization, and overall service use. Older men and women do not differ in need or use. Medical skepticism exerts some influence of utilization. A stronger belief in the value of health maintenance activities is related to use of services, suggesting the preventive health beliefs may promote use. [2.5, 12.2]

<759> White-Means, S. I., & Thornton, M. C. (1990). **Ethnic differences in the production of informal home health care.** *The Gerontologist, 30,* 758-768.

Recognizes that informal providers determine the quantity and quality of home health services received by the elderly. Conceptualizing caregiving as a type of production involving secondary caregivers assisting the primary to increase the size and productivity of caregiving systems, the authors report the need to consider ethnic diversity in this "production." In a sample of four ethnic groups, men do not make as limited a contribution to caregiving as previous research has noted, although ethnic men are no less likely to reduce their leisure time. Ethnic diversity and the organization of home care systems do recast gender effects. [9.1, 12.2, 12.3]

<760> Wingard, D. L., William-Jones, D., McPhillips, J., Kaplan, R. M., & Barrett-Conner, E. (1990). **Nursing home utilization in adults: A prospective population-based study.** *Journal of Aging and Health, 2,* 179-193.

Determines for 1,302 men and women living in an upper-middle-class community in Southern California the rates of nursing home utilization between 1972 and 1986. Leading diagnostic reasons for admission are dementia, cancer, and stroke. Rate of utilization increases with age, and men at all ages have lower utilization, although the probability of survival once admitted is lower. [11.1, 12.2, 12.3]

COMMUNITY RESOURCES AND NEEDS

<761> Berger, R. M., & Kelly, J. J. (1986). **Working with homosexuals of the older population.** *Social Casework, 67,* 203-210.

Discusses how elderly gay men are neglected by social workers and have special clinical needs. Suggests that to serve this population effectively, clinicians need to develop appropriate practice strategies. Issues unique to this population include the effects of inaccurate stereotypes, the concealment of the homosexuality from others, relationship patterns and living arrangements, and the advantages of gay aging. One damaging stereotype is that aging gays have isolated themselves from social and sexual contact and almost always live alone. In actuality, many older gays are socially and sexually active and have more variety in their living arrangements than do heterosexuals. They often have better support systems to meet the stresses of aging than do older heterosexuals. The adaptations of aging gays can provide clues as to how older individuals--both homosexual and heterosexual--facilitate their adaptation to aging. Coping with stigma, early self-reliance, role flexibility, and androgyny all appear to help the individual age well. [6.1, 12.3]

<762> Chappell, N. L. (1985). Social support and the receipt of home care services. *The Gerontologist, 25,* 47-54.

Explores differences between the elderly in Manitoba who use formal home care services and those who do not. Data are on 400 users and 400 nonusers. Analyses confirm that nonusers are more likely to be men who live in their own homes, have worked in professional or high-level management jobs, and are not widowed. Users are more likely those without social support and in need (e.g., the older and more functionally impaired). [12.2, 12.3]

<763> Choi, N. G. (1994). Patterns and determinants of social service utilization: Comparison of the childless elderly and elderly parents living with or apart from their children. *The Gerontologist, 34,* 353-362.

Analyzes the effects of the absence of children who provide important emotional and instrumental support for childless elders. Data are from the Longitudinal Survey of Aging. Childless elderly are more likely to say that they lack informal instrumental support at times of illness than are elderly parents, nevertheless the childless elderly are more likely to use social services. Older men, especially single older men, use social services more than older women. [12.3]

<764> Cohen, C. I., Teresi, J. A., Holmes, D., & Roth, E. (1988). Survival strategies of older homeless men. *The Gerontologist, 28,* 58-66.

Summarizes how one in four homeless men are 60 and older, how they are very likely not attached to public shelters and other service organizations, and how many homeless elder men periodically live on the street. Investigates the ability of homeless men (N = 281) age 50 and over from the Bowery to procure basic necessities such as money, food, shelter, and health care. Concludes that the inability to fulfill basic needs is primarily associated with the men's physical health, greater depression, lack of affiliation and contact with institutions and agencies, and stress. [10.1, 12.3]

<765> Cutler, S. J., & Coward, R. T. (1992). Availability of personal transportation in households of elders: Age, gender, and residence differences. *The Gerontologist, 32,* 77-81.

Hypothesizes that readily available transportation can enhance the quality of life of elders, providing independence and access to services, resources, and activities. Examines age and gender correlates of the availability of personal transportation in the households of elders. Using 1980 Census data, finds the availability of vehicles decreases with age, is greater for men, and is highest for rural farm and lowest for central city residents. Concludes that the benefits of personal transportation are much more available to men than to women. [12.3]

<766> Gartner, A. (1984). Widower self-help groups: A preventive approach. *Social Policy*, *14* (3), 37-38.

Some research indicates that men experience greater social isolation and loneliness in widowhood than women, and widowers are less likely to find alternative sources of support than widows. For widowers at risk, early intervention may have a significant effect upon their well-being. An number of self-help groups have been established to serve the widowed in the last 15 years, yet most of these programs are not typically directed toward men, and those men who do join often drop out. Studies of self-help groups reveal that intervention facilitate adjustment to bereavement and provide social support. Many widowers might join a self-help group if one suitable to their needs, such as an all widowers' group, existed. [7.5, 12.2, 12.3]

<767> Gwyther, L. P. (1992). Research on gender and family caregiving: Implications for clinical practice. In J. W. Dwyer & R. T. Coward (Eds.), *Gender, families, and elder care* (pp. 202-218). Newbury Park, CA: Sage Publications.

Examines the implications of the gendered nature of family care for practitioners who work with elders and their families. This chapter focuses on the need for gender-sensitive assessments of elder family care and the targeting of clinical support and intervention which may be influenced by gendered norms and expectations. [9.1, 12.3]

<768> Hornbrook, M. C., Stevens, V. J., Wingfield, D. J., Hollis, J. F., Greenlick, M. R., & Ory, M. G. (1994). Preventing falls among community-dwelling older persons: Results from a randomized trail. *The Gerontologist*, *34*, 16-23.

Reports a randomized trial of a falls prevention program that addresses home safety, exercise, and behavioral risks. The program was available to 3,182 elders who are members of a large health maintenance organization. Men age 75 and older benefit most from the intervention, which reduced the odds of falling by 0.85 during the 23-month follow-up. This is explained by the fact that older men seem more attracted to as well as have a safer experience with greater exercise. However, the intervention does not have sufficient intensity or duration to have a protective effect. [2.1, 12.2, 12.3]

<769> Kart, C. S. (1991). Variation in long-term care service use by aged blacks: Data from the Supplement on Aging. *Journal of Aging and Health*, *3*, 511-526.

Identifies patterns of long-term care service use among 1,217 black adults age 55 and older. Physician services, hospital services, and nursing home institutionalization are excluded from the analysis. Greater than one-third of the sample receive help to counter difficulties in at least one activity-in-daily-living, and greater than one-quarter receive help to deal with at least one independent-activity-in-daily-living. Older black men are less likely to receive custodial help or home management services. Most help received is unpaid and from the informal support network. [12.3]

<770> Kaye, L. W., & Applegate, J. S. (1991). **Components of a gender-sensitive curriculum model for elder caregiving: Lessons from research.** *Gerontology & Geriatrics Education, 16*, 39-56.

"Taking care" in families traditionally falls to women, who comprise two-thirds of all elder caregivers and are "closer" to their elderly relatives. Discusses how women are reaching the caregiving saturation point and how morbidity patterns mean more women than men are diagnosed with Alzheimer's disease. Responsibilities for caregiving are now falling toward husbands and other men. Summarizes a study of 152 male caregivers and how these men view themselves as nurturant and expressive, and their relationships with the care recipient as stable, positive, and satisfying. Four systems theory implications of men's motivation for caregiving and the value of reintroducing gender considerations into curriculum and training sequences conclude the essay. [9.1, 12.3]

<771> Krout, J. A., Cutler, S. J., & Coward, R. T. (1990). **Correlates of senior center participation: A national analysis.** *The Gerontologist, 30*, 72-79.

Examines the correlates of senior center participation for a national sample of 13,737 elders from the Supplement on Aging of the 1984 National Health Interview Survey. Results show that men use the center less. The significant characteristics predicting user are being female, higher levels of social interaction, decreasing income, living alone, fewer functional disabilities, and living in the suburbs. [12.3]

<772> Logan, J. R., & Spitze, G. (1994). **Informal support and the use of formal services by older persons.** *Journals of Gerontology: Social Sciences, 49*, S25-S34.

Studies older persons' use of formal services in the Albany-Schenectady-Troy area. Most services are used by only a minority of older persons. These is some evidence of both compensatory process (where family support substitutes for formal care) and bridging (where the informal network helps link the older person to services). Service users are distinguished partly by their greater functional disability and indicators of predisposition (age identity and sociability), but not gender. Older men are somewhat more likely to use home services and less likely to use community-based seniors service, but this observation is not predictive. [7.5, 12.3]

<773> Noelker, L. S., & Bass, D. M. (1989). **Home care for elderly persons: Linkages between formal and informal caregivers.** *Journals of Gerontology: Social Sciences, 44*, S63-S70.

Research predicting contact with community services has focused on characteristics of elderly persons. Investigates how community-assisted personal care and home health services are used by primary kin caretakers. Develops a typology to identify different ways caretakers take responsibility: kin independence, formal service substitution of kin, dual delivery via dual specialization, and formal system supplementing kin. Caregiver gender and relationship to the care recipient largely determine the kind of help rendered by service providers. Wives are more commonly found in the supplementation type, and husbands prefer the dual specialization type. Concludes that caregiver gender triggers different patterns of in-home service. [9.1, 12.2, 12.3]

<774> O'Brien Cousins, S., & Burgess, A. (1992). **Perspectives on older adults in physical activity and sports.** *Educational Gerontology, 18,* 461-481.

Discusses some of the difficulties facing both physical educators and older adults. Attentions is drawn to the need for educators to consider elder's gender in planning activities. Underestimation of elder's potential for learning in late life, particularly with respect to men's interests in physical activity, is very likely to reinforce stereotypes of frailty. [9.1, 12.3]

<775> Ozawa, M. N., & Morrow-Howell, N. (1992). **Service utilization by well-organized frail elderly individuals.** *International Journal of Aging and Human Development, 35,* 179-191.

Reports findings from a study of the service utilization by elders in St. Louis, Missouri. With national legislation intended to provide social services for elders, some unaddressed questions are how much elders actually use the available services and which elders use them. Finds the frail elderly are using services in greater number than prior literature has suggested. In-home services such as homemaker services and visiting nurses are used by the physically needy regardless of gender and income background; however, older women are more likely to use out-home services and transportation services, particularly those that facilitate socializing among seniors. In all, older men are not as likely to use publicly provided social services. [12.3]

<776> Rife, J. C., & First, R. J. (1989). **Discouraged older workers: An exploratory study.** *International Journal of Aging and Human Development, 29,* 195-203.

Few studies examine the impact of unemployment on the older worker. Seventy-three older unemployed workers age 50 and older who had stopped searching for a full-time job reveal a portrait of discouraged older worker as potentially at risk of both economic and psychological difficulties. Mildly depressed about their unemployment, socially isolated and embarrassed, and experiencing low life satisfaction, these unemployed workers do not reach out to social and employment-related community services. The challenges faced by the discouraged older worker suggest the need for targeted employment and supportive services to aid this population group. [2.3, 9.1, 10.2, 12.3]

<777> Schultz, C. M., & Galbraith, M. W. (1993). **Community leadership education for older adults: An exploratory study.** *Educational Gerontology, 19* (6), 473-488.

Examines the context within which older adults approach leadership roles and the processes by which they become involved in volunteer community leadership roles. Reviews a pilot program, Leadership Enhancement for the Active Retired (LEAR), which was initiated to determine if educational training in leadership would enhance the number of community leadership roles taken. The percentage of men who occupy leadership roles after taking the LEAR program was less than that of women. Results suggest four elements are associated with community leadership training: motivation, confidence building, relevance, and awareness. [12.3]

<778> Stoller, E. P., & Cutler, S. J. (1993). Predictors of use of paid help among older people living in the community. *The Gerontologist, 33,* 31-40.

Paid help is most often viewed as a supplement to the informal assistance provided by family and friends. This study examines the impact of the care-recipient's level of impairment, access to informal services, and household income to the use of paid help by impaired older people. From the Supplement on Aging to the 1984 National Health Interview Survey, finds impaired elders turn to paid help when informal services are unavailable (e.g., elder lives alone). Paid help is more prevalent among elderly people with adequate economic resources, access to entitlements, and greater need for daily personal care. Gender of care recipient does not directly affect the probability of paid help, but it likely has indirect effects by its relation to access to informal help (particularly husbands' availability of a spouse) and its effect on the decision-making process to recruit and incorporate outside support. [9.1, 12.3]

Subject Index

— ◆ —

Author Index

— ◆ —

Abelson, S., 132
Adamek, M. E., 334, 504
Adams, R. G., 439
Ade-Ridder, L., 310
Adelman, M., 69, 173
Adler, I., 634
Akiyama, H., 457, 458
Albert, M., 140, 168
Albert, S. M., 428
Aldwin, C. M., 33, 58, 63, 147, 161, 174, 181, 249, 459, 460, 644
Alecxih, L. M. B., 720
Alexander, F., 708
Allen, S. M., 70
Alterman, T., 97
Ambinder, A., 722
Ames, A., 175
Anderson, T. B., 71, 538
Andersson, L., 176
Andres, D., 98
Angel, J. L., 177
Angel, R. J., 177, 707
Anson, O., 634
Anthony-Bergstone, C. R., 559
Antonovsky, A., 634, 635
Antonovsky, H., 311
Antonucci, T. C., 457, 458, 673
Appel, J., 539
Applegate, J. S., 577, 578, 579, 770
Arber, S., 260, 560, 615, 677, 728
Arbuckle, T. Y., 98, 341
Arenberg, D., 57

Arens, D. A., 178
Arfken, C. L., 179
Armson, R. R., 103
Ashworth, J. B ., 99
Atkinson, R, M., 338
Auerbach, D., 442
Auerbach, S. M., 47
Avery, R., 517
Aviv, L., 757

Badylak, S. F., 133
Baker, J. A., 390
Baker, J. G., 207
Bar-Yam, M., 29
Barak, B.M., 1, 30, 213
Barber, H. R. K., 298
Barbre, A. R., 738
Barefoot, J. C., 68
Barer, B. M., 524
Barresi, C. M., 471, 472
Barrett-Conner, E., 100, 232, 760
Barrick, A. L., 31
Barron, K. L., 65
Bartolomei-Hill, S., 625
Barton, A, J., 466
Barusch, A. S., 561
Bass S. A., 682
Bass, D. M., 737, 773
Bastida, E., 312
Batten, H. L., 726
Bazargan, M., 738
Bearon, L. B., 750

About the Compiler

EDWARD H. THOMPSON, JR., is Associate Professor in the Department of Sociology and Anthropology, College of the Holy Cross, in Worcester, Mass. He has been actively involved as a researcher in men's studies for about a decade. Among his earlier publications are *Older Men's Lives* (1994) and numerous articles in the fields of family sociology, gerontology, and gender studies. He serves on the editorial board of *Journal of Men's Studies*.

ISBN 0-313-29106-3

90000>

EAN

9 780313 291067

HARDCOVER BAR CODE